D0763836

Growing Older

Environment and Identity in Later Life

Growing Older

Series Editor: Alan Walker

The objective of this series is to showcase the major outputs from the ESRC Growing Older programme and to provide research insights which will result in improved understanding and practice and enhanced and extended quality of life for older people.

It is well-known that people are living longer but until now very little attention has been given to the factors that determine the quality of life experienced by older people. This important new series will be vital reading for a broad audience of policymakers, social gerontologists, social policy analysists, nurses, social workers, sociologists and social geographers as well as advanced undergraduate and postgraduate students in these disciplines.

Series titles include:

Ann Bowling *Ageing Well*

Joanne Cook, Tony Maltby and Lorna Warren *Older Women's Lives*

Maria Evandrou and Karen Glaser *Family, Work and Quality of Life for Older People*

Mary Maynard, Haleh Afshar, Myfanwy Franks and Sharon Wray *Women in Later Life*

Sheila Peace, Caroline Holland and Leonie Kellaher *Environment and Identity in Later Life*

Thomas Scharf, Chris Phillipson and Allison E Smith *Ageing in the City*

Christina Victor, Sasha Scambler and John Bond *The Social World of Older People*

Alan Walker (ed.) *Growing Older in Europe*

Alan Walker and Catherine Hagan Hennessy (eds) *Growing Older: quality of life in old age*

Alan Walker (ed.) *Understanding Quality of Life in Old Age*

Growing Older

Environment and Identity in Later Life

by
Sheila Peace, Caroline Holland
and Leonie Kellaher

Open University Press

Open University Press
McGraw-Hill Education
McGraw-Hill House
Shoppenhangers Road
Maidenhead
Berkshire
England
SL6 2QL
email: enquiries@openup.co.uk
world wide web: www.openup.co.uk

and Two Penn Plaza, New York, NY 10121-2289, USA

First published 2006

Copyright © Sheila Peace, Caroline Holland and Leonie Kellaher 2006

All rights reserved. Except for the quotation of short passages for the purposes of criticism and review, no part of this publication may be reproduced, stored in a retrieval system, or transmitted, in any form, or by any means, electronic, mechanical, photocopying, recording or otherwise, without the prior permission of the publisher or a licence from the Copyright Licensing Agency Limited. Details of such licences (for reprographic reproduction) may be obtained from the Copyright Licensing Agency Ltd of 90 Tottenham Court Road, London, W1T 4LP.

A catalogue record of this book is available from the British Library

ISBN: 0 335 21511 4 (pb), 0 335 21512 2 (hb)
ISBN-13: 978 0335 21511 9 (pb), 978 0335 21512 6 (hb)

Library of Congress Cataloging-in-Publication Data
CIP data applied for

Typeset by YHT Ltd, London
Printed in the UK by Bell & Bain Ltd, Glasgow

Contents

List of figures and tables

Figures

Tables

1

Placing the self

Introduction

Does where you are affect who you are? If so, does this relationship change in later life? This book is about placing the self in later life and the interaction between environment and identity. A wide range of issues are raised: personal, family and housing histories; decisions over lifestyle and living arrangements, sometimes compensating for individual frailties; environmental press; community involvement; attachments to various places and the impact of cultural change; routines of daily living; engagement and disengagement related to comfort, security and autonomy. These are reflections from the lives of people whose life course has spanned much of the 20th century and they are themes that will be developed throughout this book as we hear from older people living in semi-rural, urban and metropolitan parts of middle and southeast England who contributed to research from 1999 to 2003 for the project, 'Environment and Identity in Later Life: A cross-setting study'.

We set out to understand the relationship between environment and identity in later life and we begin this chapter by introducing these concepts and reviewing some of the main theoretical and methodological developments in environmental gerontology. The dynamic between person and place varies but in later life we recognize two important factors: first, as people age their spatial experience may change. Many people experience long-term and recent frailties that can influence everyday decisions about activities. However, while physical frailty and personal competence are related they should not be seen as synonymous. In spite of poor health a majority of people maintain routines and find ways of supporting them for as long as possible. Second, older people bring the experience of time to this dynamic. This research therefore confronts issues of continuity and change in time and space and in this sense our analysis has to be biographical, generational, historical and contemporary – themes to be found threaded throughout the rich narratives that form this study.

To begin we need to define environment and identity. These are two very well-researched topics that, on first thought, may prompt us to relate 'identity' to the disciplines of psychology and sociology and 'environment' to geography (physical and social), psychology, ecology, planning, architecture, engineering. As researchers the authors are a multidisciplinary team influenced by anthropology, human geography, sociology, social policy, environmental psychology, history and gerontology. We begin by setting out the theoretical influences that have guided our study and that our own ongoing work build on in the area of environment and ageing (see Peace et al., 1982, 1997, 2005; Willcocks et al., 1987; Hanson et al., 2001; Peace and Holland, 2001; Kellaher, 2002).

Reflections on identity in later life

To most people, identity relates to how they see themselves, which will impact on how they react to what is happening around them and what they reflect back to other people. How we understand ourselves may relate to factors that are biological, hereditary, historical, situational, social, sexual, educational and environmental. These will affect how we appear, behave, relate to others, and influence the roles that we chose or experience in life (Burkitt, 1992; Wetherall, 1996; Holloway, 2000). We can make a distinction between self-identity and social identity. Most people, whatever their age and situation, will have a 'core' or an 'essence' that is unique to them and others will see as them 'being themselves' – a 'self-identity'. But a personal identity also reflects a life history that is both individual and social. For example, a man of 80 years living in 2001, who was born in England to British parents, is likely to have had experience of World War Two. This experience, which will be similar in some ways for all people of his generation, and compounded by additional similarities for people of the same gender, culture, ethnicity or similar social class, creates a 'social identity'. In stressing commonalities, social identities can lead to stereotypes although experience is inevitably different for each person due to unique life histories.

Where we are and who we are with will affect our behaviour; our sense of well-being and how we think about ourselves. Personal strengths and weaknesses which contribute to self-identity can be exposed as people juxtapose different social roles and it is this constant rebalancing that may make people appear to have identities that are not fixed. The development of social roles (e.g. familial, paternal, managerial) will relate to individual characteristics/personalities, varying in type and possessing different meanings that will change over time. To this understanding of identity we add the domain of environment – the context in which people encounter self in later life and that is reflected back to others: a situated identity (Hockey and James, 2003). Knowing who we are, 'being able to read ourselves', will help us to weather the range of different situations in which we find ourselves.

Life experiences influence identity and across the life course those experiences will be crucially formative. American gerontologists Rubinstein and Parmelee defined identity in later life in this way:

> [I]dentity is the sense of who one is in the world, distilled from a lifetime of experiences. From the collective perspective, identity consists of the life course as a cultural construct: socially normative and collectively outlined and accepted life course statuses and transitions. But at the individual level, every person creates for herself a particularized version of the collective life course, a life story, depending upon her specific experiences and the meaning she attaches to them. (1992, p.144)

Here they consider 'accepted life course statuses and transitions' as affecting the 'cultural construct' of identity. This view led us to reconsider the ongoing work of lifespan developmental psychologists. Can developmental stages influence how people perceive their own identity and does this relate at all to how people interact with their environment? We returned to Erikson, pioneer in research into personality development, who presented a framework for discussing the cumulative impact of different life stages (Erikson, 1965). He positioned the emergence of identity and role confusion within youth as individuals become concerned with 'what they appear to be in the eyes of others'; whereas in considering later life his thoughts turned to differing levels of engagement and acceptance. He saw the last phase of life as a time of 'ego integrity' – a sense of meaning and order in life that could be set against 'despair' due to a failure to accept life's path. He commented that 'integrity' involves 'the acceptance of one's one and only life cycle as something that had to be and that, by necessity, permitted of no substitution' (1965, p.260). While later writings recognized how cultural difference and the complexity of changing circumstances may affect these outcomes, impeding or encouraging the development of full potential (Erikson, 1982; Erikson et al., 1986; Coleman, 1993a), this comment also recognizes the exchange between the person and their environment. Consequently, while considered as stages the issues discussed are cumulative and experienced uniquely. As Bond et al. comment:

> The emphasis on integrity of the lifespan is Erikson's lasting contribution and one that is vital to an understanding of old age. In order to understand people in late life it is necessary to see them in the context of their whole life history with the problems both successfully and unsuc- cessfully resolved from earlier periods of life. This approach to human development and human ageing contains a number of important implications. The first is that the situations of older individuals will vary according to their histories. The courses of development of different people are likely to diverge the longer they live, and the more experiences they absorb. Rather than growing more alike as we age, we therefore become more individual. (1993, pp.29–30)

These comments have a particular resonance for this study and its methodological approach. There has been an important recognition of the constant interchange between the individual and their environ- mental and social circumstances that can lead to continued growth through maintaining expertise and control, and developing new skills that will support morale. However, there has also been recognition that even within a society that recognizes itself as ageing, negative ageist values may compound this engagement through personal losses, leading to low self-esteem and a consequent impact on self-identity.

The late 20th century has seen the work of other social scientists concerned with the self in later life and research concerning personality indicates levels of variation between people in terms of introversion/ extroversion – from those who become more preoccupied with their inner self, to those who remain mentally engaged with the outside world (Sugarman, 1986; Gutmann, 1987; Baltes and Baltes, 1990; Coleman, 1993b; Baltes and Carstensen, 1996; Baltes and Mayer, 1999; Smith et al., 1999). Old age is seen to involve different adaptive processes as people with a variety of somatic and socioeconomic circumstances cope or do not cope (Staudinger et al., 1999). The Berlin Aging Study (BASE) 1999 has shown that adaptive capacity may be more limited among people of advanced old age (85+) and that both this group and persons living in institutions reported less frequent experience of positive emotions (Smith et al., 1999). They also found mainly age-associated differences in social activities and social participation, both of which are highly related to health status (Mayer et al., 1999). In considering the influence of age on identity we would argue that while they may be situated differently, older people are just as or even more strategic than younger people in constructing identity.

Changing times and places

The life course of any individual takes place within changing times and research involving older people with ages ranging from 93 to 61 years, born between 1907 and 1939, needs to acknowledge generational experience. While the former may have been involved in World War Two, the latter would have been war babies, becoming young adults during the 1960s. We may expect the relationship between life stage and identity formation to be intimately entwined but in recent years this has been questioned (Giddens, 1991). Ageing societies in western developed countries are changing rapidly, leading to diversity in the construction of individual identity in the 'postmodern' world. Individual experience has become less controlled by overarching social structures and institutions such as the church, the family and the nation state. Instead, society has become increasingly individualistic and concerned with modes of consumption where people face a multitude of choices. A plethora of available lifestyles has led to ontological insecurity and to the exclusion of those groups without the resources to participate (Askham, 2002). These are all concerns that make the contextualization of self within later life more important than has perhaps been realized to date.

How do people actively develop and adopt ideas and meanings

about themselves and sustain them in relation to the challenges, complexities and anxieties of life? In times of change, Giddens (1991) has raised the importance of globalization in the development of self-identity, stating:

> The self is not a passive entity, determined by external influences; in forging their self-identities, no matter how local their specific contexts of action, individuals contribute to and directly promote social influences that are global in their consequences and implications. (1991, p.2)

This quote juxtaposes the self against globalizing influences noting the reflexivity that occurs with continuous change as action/behaviour at a micro level influences broader societal trends that influence individual action and so on. In outlining his arguments regarding 'modernity and self-identity', Giddens highlights how modern social life can involve the reorganization of time and space. They are no longer dependent on each other but can mix and match in infinite possibilities, e.g. the video conference; the 24-hour drive-in restaurant; the TV viewing of lifestyles in different parts of the world. He sees modernity as post-traditional where the 'sureties of tradition and habit' are replaced by features of 'doubt' and 'risk' and where 'trust' forms the path to ontological security in that it allows for a confidence/mastery of action even where there is no certainty. In this way, he recognizes context as influential in supporting personal autonomy over everyday routines in what may now be called the postmodern world. Using these ideas we question whether 'trust' through attachment to place in later life leads to a sense of security and how retaining mastery through engagement and re-engagement enables people to cope with both staying in place or moving. But first how do we define and understand environment or the context of living?

Layered environment

Important authors from a range of disciplines have written influentially on space, time and identity (e.g. Soja, 1989; Massey, 1994; Pile and Thrift, 1995). In particular, Goffman (1959, 1961) has been concerned with how people relate to each other within a wide range of situations both communal and institutional. His concern with how people present themselves to others led him to use perspectives from theatrical performance to aid understanding. Spatially, he defined front and back regions where different versions of 'self' could be portrayed. Bourdieu (1977) examined the material culture of everyday life to analyze how this is employed in the construction of individual practices and habits. In developing the concept of 'habitus', he concentrated on the domestic setting and its materialities. However, while time is implicated in the evolution of customs etc. at individual and collective levels, he does not comment on age-distinctive patterns (Bourdieu, 1977). Others, notably, Lefebvre (1991) have argued for the ways in which people – at any age – live and make sense of a changing world and how past, present and future are constructed through spatial and temporal frames. This theme also underpins the body of work by cultural geographers in unpacking the subjectivity of the spatial imperative (Longhurst, 2003).

In the late 1990s, the geographer Laws was particularly interested in the spatiality of ageing from a structural perspective. She viewed the ageism of space where 'youth is everywhere and older people invisible' (1997) and used the development of age-segregated communities and housing to consider the links between social processes and spatial arrangements in society. She saw identity as 'constantly renegotiated' and argued that identities could be imposed by external forces such as ageist, racist or sexist stereotypes or developed through internal forces – the internalization of stereotypes – commenting that 'Where we are says a lot about who we are' (1997, p.93). She argued that there are a number of spatial factors that can affect the identity of older people and lead to their inclusion or exclusion in society including:

- *accessibility* to particular places (nation state; residential neighbourhood; workplace), which can affect a person's citizenship status and consequently their identity

- *mobility* both metaphorical and material, between places and social situations – a marker of your social position relative to others

- *motility* – the body's 'potential' to move – can lead to the labelling of frailty, which has an impact on public identity

- *spatial scale* – how older people are seen within different social groups from the domestic to the national (loving grandparent to the 'burden' of old people)

♦ *spatial segregation* – produced by limitations just outlined, which can lead to social control of a group.
(developed from Laws, 1997, p.93)

She considers how changing aged identities can result in changing spatial environments – a form of 'discursive identity' that can be seen in both the material and representational environment. To demonstrate this argument she considers how the separation of generations between households has changed the domestic built environment and how institutionalization can represent the negative burden of ageing. She suggests that the experience of being old varies according to environment, arguing that space can mediate or constrain personal experience. In considering age-segregated communities she argues that location is important in spatially segregating older people from city life, which nonetheless remains within reach.

Environmental complexity

Our consideration of these texts led us to reflect on the other central component of our study – environment – which in general we take to mean both the place and space that encompass the person and affect their understanding of themselves and the culture in which they live. We have identified a number of definitional levels that have been confirmed through our data. First, we can distinguish macro and micro environments. We are concerned with aspects of life that may be experienced as global, international, national, regional or local. These we define as *macro environments* diversely experienced whose status may be administrative, symbolic or public – beyond the familial, domestic or intimate world but influencing the creation of self-identity through spatiality. In contrast, we see *micro environments* as encompassing the habitat, the place of living, accommodation, the immediate surroundings of the individual and the metaphysical environment. These two levels will, of course, overlap, for each subject will inhabit the micro within the macro simultaneously.

The linking of these two environmental levels brings us to the second definition, which sees the understanding of environment as linked to physical (natural/material), social and psychological facets that may be examined separately but seen as intimately connected. The *physical environment* includes both the *natural* environment – wild and cultivated – and the *material* environment that has been built, designed and placed within a specific space. The design of buildings and public spaces shape different places and affect the relationships that people have with each other. The *social environment* reflects the way in which people utilize their social capital to occupy, use and organize their surroundings, impacting on their behaviour with others and this may influence the *psychological environment* – the meaning of place and space and the emotionality that different people feel in their attachment to environment, however experienced.

A number of commentators suggest they move between these layers and this is the mechanism where named 'place' is derived from use of 'space'. Here we find our third understanding of environment as – *public, private* and *personal*. Space is all around us but the subjectivity of space into place, that makes it public, private or personal, is found in the way in which boundaries are set around or within to determine territoriality, accessibility and usage. Literature exploring the use of space shows how behaviour may be influenced by cultural, social and individual practices (Sommer, 1969; Altman and Low, 1992; Veitch and Arkkelin, 1995; Probyn, 2003). For example: access to a space around the body can change depending on intimacy and familiarity, affecting privacy (Twigg, 1999); religious practice may influence how men and women use space for socialization (National Federation of Housing Associations, 1993). In these instances, the meaning of space relates to the ways in which people use and have access to it and accessibility may have different rules, customs and practices relating to issues of control and surveillance.

Unpacking the complex meaning of environment we can identify terms such as 'context', 'milieu', 'surroundings', 'settings', 'accommodation', 'neighbourhood' and 'home range' defined in relation to a specific situation or role; a sense of atmosphere; an attachment to place, or the ability of a 'area of comfort' to maintain and develop well-being. The research discussed in this text began with a recognition that environment could have any of these meanings for the research respondents. We did not know how they would define environment or convey its impact on their own identity; we expected interpretations to emerge and we could see that environment has potential to be layered.

Nevertheless, as researchers we pragmatically defined environment in two ways: through the choice of *locations* (metropolitan, urban and semi-rural) within middle and southeast England 1999–2002; and a determination to include respondents living in *accommodation* that could be called *'ordinary' housing* – available to any person and age integrated – and *'special' housing* – specifically developed for older people and therefore age segregated. To date, little research undertaken in the UK involves older people living in this range of accommodation within one study. Research into the lives of older people living in all forms of 'special' housing has been more extensive (for example, see Townsend, 1962; Willcocks et al., 1987; Peace et al., 1997; Oldman and Quilgars, 1999; Mozley et al., 2004) than 'ordinary' housing (Oldman, 1990; Means, 1997; Peace and Holland, 2001; Heywood et al., 2002; Sumner, 2002) as funding bodies have been keen to evaluate aspects of accommodation and care. By including a cross-section of environments that can offer different levels of informal and formal support it becomes possible to comment on the ways in which people address the changing relationship between environment and self-identity until close to the end of their lives.

Oral historian Bornat (1998), discussing identity and life experience, raises a number of questions regarding the ongoing formation of self and social identity that can also be related to this topic: 'Do you have a sense of your particular place within the flow of life going on around you?' 'Has the meaning that you have about yourself changed over time?' 'Has the meaning been evolved through the relationships that you have had with others – is it socially constructed?' To which we add: 'Does your experience of environment tell us something about you?' Such questions have been and continue to be asked by those interested in the ageing of society. Before considering our own research we turn to this literature.

Theoretical links between environment, identity and age

In reviewing recent European literature, gerontologists interested in environment and ageing have focused on the lives of older people in different situations; from British research on the meaning of home (Sixsmith, 1986; 1990; Gurney and Means, 1993; Chapman and Hockey, 1999); to discussions of the village community in rural Finland (Koskinen and Outila, 2002); to understanding the development of shared living in Co Housing in Denmark and the Netherlands (BiC, 1994; Jones, 1997; VROM, 1997); to the implications of migration in later life both within and between countries (Warnes, 1991; 2004).

Considering this broad sweep of research prompts reflection on the theoretical development that has influenced this research and underpins our own (see Peace et al., 1982, 1997; Willcocks et al., 1987). The roots of environment and ageing research lie in the work of North American and European urban sociologists, ecologists and psychologists of the 1920s and 1930s (Park et al., 1925; Lewin, 1936; Murray, 1938). Murray first used the term 'press' to distinguish the way in which personal development could be related to the type of context in which people were situated. This early body of work underpins later theoretical development by gerontologists – primarily psychologists, anthropologists and geographers – whose work from the 1960s onwards on ecology and ageing; spatiality in later life; and attachment to place has been influential in developing this field from the perspective of the individual (see Peace et al., 2005).

Ecology of ageing

> [A] person's behavioural and psychological state can be better understood with knowledge of the context in which the person behaves. (Lawton, 1980, p.2)

The words of psychologist Powell Lawton concern the way in which the individual copes with a particular situation at a point in time. In 1968, Lawton and Simon developed the *'environmental docility hypothesis'* which stated that: 'The less competent the individual, the greater the impact of environmental factors on that individual' (1980, p.14). This was further developed in the ecological model of Lawton and Nahemow (1973), known as the press-competence model, which introduced the concept of *environmental press*. Here individual competence could be considered within the immediate and wider environments in which a person lived, enabling a judgement on the degree of comfort and performance potential that could be experienced. Their views were based on research carried out with vulnerable older people and 'competence' was defined as 'the theoretical upper limit of capacity of the individual to function in the areas of biological health, sensation and perception, motor behaviour and cognition' (Lawton, 1983, p.350)

11

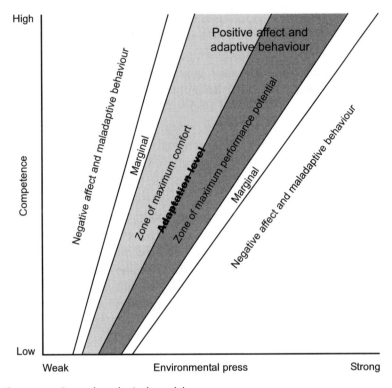

Figure 1.1 General ecological model
Source: Lawton and Nahemow, 1973

assessed through measurable tasks (Rubinstein and De Medeiros, 2004). Central to the model was an adaptation level where people were able to '*tune out the environment*' (see Figure 1.1) (Lawton, 1980, p.13, 2000, pp.190–191) by achieving a state of balance between the comfort zone and the challenge zone. While acknowledging that the environment did have meaning, this was not the central focus of this research.

However, Lawton's understanding of environment was complex and multifaceted, ranging from the characteristics of housing and the age mix of a neighbourhood to the impact of societal structures such as legislative regulations (Lawton, 1980). He saw linkages across the varied aspects of the micro and macro environments (Lawton, 1999) although this level of complexity was underdeveloped within his research (Wahl and Lang, 2004). It was through environmental press that the individual became aware of their environment and this could occur at both macro and micro levels. For example, neighbourhood change could present a form of 'press' within the external environment, while a change of health status could lead a person to experience a housing environment as disabling.

Environmental press could also be seen as a stimulus leading to problem solving or 'environmental pro-activity' (Lawton, 1989), and how an older person coped with this change would relate to personal competence and whether they can either adapt their behaviour in order to maintain their well-being, or adapt the environment to make it more manageable. Indeed, adaptation can become something that people do all the time, albeit unconsciously. The initial definition of competence did not encompass a sense of growth; rather it was more associated with a decline in competence. However, in later work both Lawton (1999) and Nahemow (2000) considered the fluidity of health and illness and consequent changes in competence and recognized limitations in using competence to assess interactions with the environment. Alongside Lawton, other American researchers were also exploring person/environment fit. The work of Kahana and Kahana (1983), Carp and Carp (1984) and Carp (1987, 1994), within both institutional settings and community locations, has focused on how a misfit between person and environment could become detrimental even to someone using their full potential; seen in both psychological as well as physical characteristics such as motivations and needs.

The perspective of person/environment fit is central to many areas of environmental research. In the UK, a recent development of this approach can be seen in multidisciplinary research, particularly between architectural, engineering, computing and social science disciplines, seeking to understand how older people may cope with environmental press in terms of the material/physical environment through the aid of assistive technology (Fisk, 2001; Marshall, 2001; McCreadie and Tinker, 2005). Yet, as noted earlier, environment is a complex topic and the present research empowers older people to define environment for themselves. Interactions between the material, the social and the psychological environments will be noted and there are still areas where too little is known; for example, the importance of being part of a couple in preventing or delaying environmental press is a topic raised in this research. It is therefore unsurprising that recent critiques of the literature comment on the need to unpack this complexity:

> [T]he basic insights of the empirical literature support that both the social and physical environment form the 'context' of aging, but the relations and interfaces between these are mostly ignored as a conceptual challenge. (Wahl and Lang, 2004, p.6)

With this critique in mind, we consider the work of authors who have taken an approach to research in this area that focuses on the subjective individual.

Subjective experiences of ageing in place

The social geographer Graham Rowles and anthropologist Robert Rubenstein represent gerontologists who have developed ethnographic methodologies that allow detailed analysis of the lives of older people in context. From the late 1970s onwards Rowles has developed a theoretical perspective on the geographical experience of older people in terms of both space and place. His seminal study, *Prisoners of Space* (1978), used detailed biographical material from five older people to develop a framework examining four areas of experience: activity, orientation, feeling and fantasy. These four areas embraced complexity by covering activities across the widest range of spatial cognition including the metaphysical. Each topic incorporates the detail of daily living, mapping out the varying levels of experience. For example, *activity* could include movements between rooms within a house as well as less frequent visits to a friend.

Figure 1.2 outlines the scope defined by *orientation*. Orientation relates to an awareness of place that may be hierarchical (proximate or distant) but is constantly reordered in terms of meaning. The cognition of space is also associated with behaviour, which can affect how possessive a person feels about and acts toward a place.

Emotional attachment to place is an important part of personal experience for many people and part of what we have called the psychological environment. Here Rowles defines *feelings* as having differing levels of permanence and association with people and events. The degree of permanence may vary from emotions that relate to immediate reactions to temporary feelings that come and go, to more permanent attachments. Rowles also relates emotions to the social

---

Orientation – relates to an understanding or cognition of space

> *Personal schema* – facility to direct action within 'lived space'
>
> *Specific schemata* – paths, routes, nodes used to negotiate the environment and facilitating orientation in different circumstances, e.g. seasonal, temporal, gradational
>
> *General schema* – related to experientially distinctive domains embedded within each other:
>
> > *Home* – the fulcrum
> >
> > *Surveillance zone* – field of vision from the home, not inviolable space but watchful space
> >
> > *Neighbourhood* – functionally defined but with experiential boundaries, social affinity identification threatened by neighbourhood transition
> >
> > *City* – more fragmented and disjointed differentiation of space; separate from local; known through personal history; individual settings within wider spatial entity; affection plus transitions
> >
> > *'Beyond space'* – significant locations

Figure 1.2 Orientation
Source: Developed from Rowles, 1978, pp. 157–203

environment through associations that may relate to individual experience or to a communality of feeling shared by others.

Finally, he turns to the places of imagination and recollection which he calls *fantasy*, commenting that: 'Fantasies are creative "grand fictions" through which the individual moulds a separate personal reality' (1978, p.180). In this sense he stresses the great significance that he feels is played by participation in both past and displaced contemporary settings. This metaphysical environment is unique to the individual and can be liberating, sometimes prompted by contextual cues through artefacts, pictures, media.

By exploring these four aspects of geographical experience, Rowles considers that quality of life may be supported where personal capabilities and environmental opportunity are balanced through ongoing adjustments (1978, p.190). Such a study was ambitious. In later work he has continued to explore aspects of this framework in greater depth, particularly within rural environments, developing the concept of 'insideness', which he suggests has three attributes:

- *physical insideness* – familiarity with the physical setting

- *social insideness* – integration with the social fabric of community and possible age peer group culture

- *autobiographical* insideness – based on time and space, a historical legacy of life lived within a particular environment.

Consequently, he addresses aspects of person/environment fit, where someone has a sense of 'being in place' that draws on a life time of experience (Rowles, 1983, 1991, 2000; Rowles and Watkins, 2003; Rowles et al., 2004).

The second body of work of influence to our research is that of Rubinstein, a longtime colleague of Lawton. Here we focus on Rubenstein's work relating to how people in later life attribute meaning to the home environment and the development of attachment to place. In 1989 Rubinstein published a detailed study of the micro environment of the home based on detailed ethnographic research with seven older Americans, which he describes in this way:

> After an initial meeting, when the goals of the project were explained, each subject was visited by the author once a week, at his or her home for most of a morning or afternoon, for approximately four months ... . Visits often consisted of a regular, formal, open-ended interview, chitchat, and in some instances helping with chores. Data, consisting of responses, commentary, and observations of behaviour at home, were recorded longhand during or immediately after the interview meeting and were coded on the basis of emerging topics and personal issues. Such review and categorization in turn helped in formulating additional questions for the ongoing interviews. (1989, p.S46)

He adopted a psychosocial approach seeing older people as proactive in creating personal meaning through aspects of their subjective world such as objects, rooms, furniture and routines and describes three classes of empirically derived psychosocial processes as 'standards of personhood':

+ *'social-centred processes'* – relating to sociocultural order

+ *'person-centred processes'* – relating to the life course

+ *'body-centred processes'* – relating to the body.

Each of these processes was derived through analysis of the ongoing discussions. In Rubinstein's view, sociocultural order concerns processes that link person to place through the 'correct way of doing things'; shared notions of correct standards and behaviour; the ordering of space; the proper times and places for particular activities – which became the *social-centred* processes. In relation to *person-centred processes*, he focused on how the environment comes to embody a person's life course and considered four elements of place attachment through personalization involving increasing degrees of identification with objects in the environment from those that are just identified to those which come to represent self. He comments:

> [E]mbodiment can be important to some older people for whom, at the current time, aspects of the physical environment may have a potential for greater endurance than their own bodies. Environmental features may therefore be assigned the task, through embodiment, of carrying the load of personal meaning and thereby aid in the maintenance of self, when it is threatened. (1989, p.S50)

Finally, in terms of the body, he described two processes: *entexturing*, where regulation of the environment serves to induce a sensory state of comfort; and *environmental centralization*, so that the environment is manipulated over time to accommodate increasing limitations of the body. Peripheral areas of the home are closed off and living space is concentrated into central zones: less important activities are abandoned to muster energy for those that are felt to be important. In considering these three psychosocial processes Rubinstein begins to address how personhood can be seen within environment, recognizing that such processes may also be reconstructed following changes in environment.

Further development of this work is seen in the early 1990s. Rubinstein and Parmelee (1992) viewed attachment behaviour as a life-course phenomenon concerning place as lived currently and in memory. Their discussion of place attachment has resonance with that of Rowles, outlining the way in which space may become place:

> Personal experience, either direct or vicarious ... and social interaction lead the person to attach meaning to a defined space; as a result, within his or her own identity, it becomes a place. (1992, p.142)

In addition, they raise the important relationship between time and space in establishing the meaning of place and argue that: 'The very notion of place implies a conflation of space and time such that attachment to a particular place may also represent attachment to a particular time' (1992, p.142) and in earlier work Rubinstein argued that this attachment may be 'strong or weak', 'positive or negative', 'narrow, wide or diffuse' (1990).

Rubinstein and Parmelee present an 'integrative model of place attachment in late life' and argue that this is understood through three essential elements: *geographic behaviour*, *identity* and *interdependence*. These encompass the locational and social life of the individual, which provides for the 'dialectic of autonomy and security' seen as the major environmental theme of old age (Parmelee and Lawton, 1990). The three elements are viewed as spanning two dimensions: *the collective* (i.e. the meanings inherent to a given culture and shared by its members) and *the individual* (i.e. meanings derived from personal attitudes, beliefs and experiences) and they argue that there are three reasons why place attachment is important to older people:

* keeping the past alive

* remaining constant during times of change

* maintaining a sense of continued competence.

The importance of this work is seen in bringing together the 'significance of objective place characteristics and subjective place experiences', which parallels the work of Rowles. It has been central to our understanding of the interface of material, social and psychological environment and provides an underpinning to this study.

Current developments

In more recent years the field of environmental gerontology has become interdisciplinary leading to multi-method research and European scholars are beginning to critique and extend the North American dominance of this field. For example, in the late 20th century the EU-funded ENABLE-AGE project brought together gerontologists and practitioners from the disciplines of psychology, sociology, primary care and occupational therapy to consider '*the home environment as a determinant for autonomy, participation, and well-being in very old age in a longitudinal perspective, exploring subjective and objective aspects of housing and their impact on health and ageing*' within five European countries: Sweden, Germany, the United Kingdom, Hungary and Latvia.[1] An ambitious study, the project includes both large-scale surveys with very old people living alone in private urban homes with a follow-up design, comprising two measurement points with a one-year interval, and in-depth qualitative interviews with a smaller number of respondents. While the researchers are developing their own project-specific conceptual framework, they have drawn on Lawton's ecological model and the WHO's work on disability functioning (ICF). The research has used and developed a wide range of measures concerning subjective and objective issues from housing standards to the meaning of home assessing the impact for the individual through medical, psychological, social and community perspectives. They aim to develop a methodology that could be used in individual case management regarding housing decisions. The extensive nature of that study reflects the level of complexity that is also seen in this study.

Ways forward

All these authors have influenced our work, which develops, expands and challenges some of their ideas and theoretical and conceptual developments. While recent comment by Phillipson (2004) have drawn attention to the need for environmental gerontologists to address postmodern societal issues of globalization and urbanization, this study seeks an understanding of the experience of these changes through the eyes of individuals living in differing locations and situations. How then have we developed our methodological approach? A number of questions arose. Given the focus on environment and identity – how has age, life history, gender, culture impacted on life–place choices? Does increasing age lead to marginalization in place and space as raised by Laws (1997)? Is this still the case for retired 'amenity-migrant' migrant two-homers whose financial resources may support their autonomy until an advanced age; or for the long timer who has lived in the same house for 40 years and become part of neighbourhood life? Our concern is environment and identity. While the materiality of accommodation is important this may not be the central focus. Is visibility important to identity? Reflections on our own earlier research within age-segregated environments led us to realize that the need for diversity in terms of both location and living environment, both age integrated and age segregated, was crucial for the present study. We needed to talk to people who lived in a range of settings and places. Consequently, in order to contextualize the research we need to consider where British older people live.

Older people's housing in the UK

Throughout the 20th century and on into the 21st both the proportions and absolute number of people over the age of 65 years in Britain has continued to grow (Glaser and Tomassini, 2002). By 2031 over one-third of the population in England and Wales will be over 65 years and the proportions within the older age groups will continue to increase from 9.5% being 75 plus in 2001 to 13.8% in 2031.[2] Given an ageing society, it becomes important to recognize the inclusivity of groups through age and the way in which such inclusion may be demonstrated spatially. Examination of census data shows that those areas of the UK with the highest proportion of people of post-retirement age are concentrated in Wales, Cornwall and coastal districts of southwest England with densities also in the southeast and northeast. The areas with low proportions of older people include Northern Ireland and London, although in metropolitan areas there is greater cultural diversity of this population. As can be seen from Figure 1.3, given variation in population density, people spend their later years in urban, suburban and semi-rural areas, locational effects reflected in this study.

To complement location, an examination of living arrangements is essential (see Table 1.1) and through an examination of a range of data from the *British Household Panel Survey*, the *General Household Survey*, the *Survey of English Housing*, the *British Social Attitudes Survey*,[3] Glaser and Tomassini (2002, pp.76–95) identify a number of trends in the late 20th/early 21st centuries:

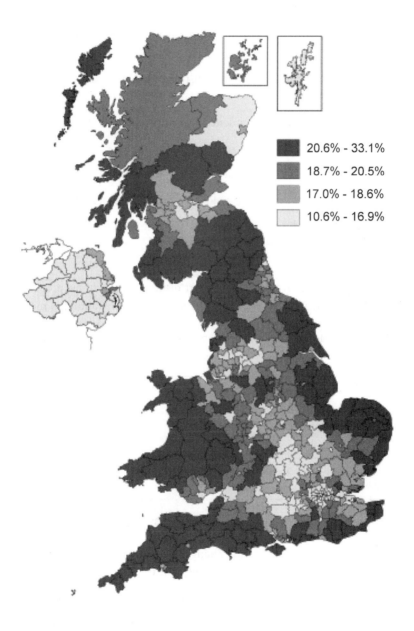

Figure 1.3 Geographic distribution of people over pensionable age
Source: Census, April 1991, Office for National Statistics; Census, April 2001, General Register Office for Scotland; Census, April 2001, Northern Ireland Statistics and Research Agency; Census, April 2001, Office for National Statistics

◆ An increase in the proportion of older people living alone, especially women.

◆ A decline in the number living with relatives, particularly children, or the non-related.

◆ Greater residential independence and 'intimacy at a distance'.

◆ Recent increase in older people living as couples.

◆ Continued increase in unmarried older women living alone.

◆ Most of the care received by older people is from family members.

◆ A majority of older people do not migrate or want to move and high levels of housing satisfaction are reported (Warnes, 1996; Glaser et al., 1998).

◆ Those who do move travel only short distances and women are more likely than men to give health and family reasons for wanting to move.

Table 1.1 Trends in living arrangements of older people aged 65+: General Household Survey, 1998

Living arrangement	Men	Women
	1998 (%)	
Living alone	23.3	45.6
Couple only	64.6	40.6
Couple and children only	5.3	2.1
Other	6.8	11.7
Total N=	**1412**	**1824**

Source: Adapted from Glaser and Tomassini, 2002, p.85

Central to this analysis are changes in survivorship and marital status and two important contrasting features appear to impact in different ways on couples and singles. The greater life expectancy of women in relation to men has been narrowing in recent years leading to an increase in the percentage of those choosing marriage or partnership, living as couples (Murphy and Grundy, 1994; Grundy, 1996, 1999; Glaser, 1997). At the same time, 'solo living' is currently of particular relevance for women of advanced age and research shows that future cohorts reaching very old age in the 2020s and 2030s are more likely to be lone householders (Evandrou and Falkingham, 2000). These changes have the potential to impact on how people in the future will view different forms of housing in later life (Peace forthcoming, 2006).

But in what type of accommodation are people currently living? The great majority (approximately 85%) of people over retirement age live in mainstream age-integrated housing. The English House Conditions Survey identifies eight categories of housing type:

- purpose-built, high-rise flat

- purpose-built, low-rise flat

- converted flat

- bungalow

- detached house

- semi-detached house

- medium–large terraced

- small terraced. (Source: DETR (1998))

Kellaher (2002, p.40) comments that older people are most likely to live in bungalows, low-rise purpose-built flats – both likely to be sheltered housing across different tenures – and though numbers are small detached houses. In terms of tenure, data from the General Household Survey for 2000–2001 (ONS, 2002) show that 53% of households over pensionable age owned their property outright whereas 35% rented in the social sector; the remainder either owned with a mortgage or rented privately.

Communal settings that are to different degrees age segregated offer accommodation and care services through sheltered housing, extra-care housing and care homes. The numbers of older people living and dying in these different types of accommodation varies with age. Heywood et al. (2002) comment:

> The numbers of older people living in communal living arrangements is small. Around 5 per cent of people aged 65 or over in Britain lived in sheltered housing in 1994 and a further 5 percent lived in housing with a non-resident warden (Tinker et al., 1999). Around 5 percent of all older people aged over 65, but 20 per cent of those over 85, live in residential care homes, nursing homes or hospital.

In recent years extra-care housing, currently accommodating 20,000 older people, has been developed to satisfy the need for lifelong housing (Laing, 2005). The variation in population and popularity found in these types of accommodation with care reflects their historical development (see Peace et al., 1997; Heywood et al., 2002) and the rhetoric regarding housing and home as a symbol of personal identity and self. A key issue is the fact that in sheltered and extra-care housing you have 'your own front door', a boundary of control and privacy.

The ownership of communal establishments may be public, private-for-profit or voluntary not-for-profit and residents, predominantly women, may be tenants or owners. The lifestyles of this range of people vary enormously from those for whom the environment allows for independent living to those in great need of assistance. People living within care homes can be extremely frail and in a recent study based in 30 British care homes, Mozley et al. (2004, pp.69/70) show that 64% of recently admitted residents had severe or very severe cognitive impairment and that depression was also common; factors affecting the need for assistance with activities of daily living and, consequently, the level of organizational infrastructure.

Research approach and methodology

An understanding of this national picture is an essential background to a study concerned with the interface between environment and identity in later life. It points this research in three directions: *first*, to recognize the need to include people living in both mainstream and age-segregated housing and accommodation with care;[4] *second*, to include a range of housing types and tenures; and *third*, to recognize the importance of location incorporating a diversity of community types from urban to rural. Having determined these prerequisites, a methodology was sought to answer the key question posed by this research: *How far can the layered environment be drawn on to reflect the complex self in later life?*

The research design outlined here was underpinned by a conviction that the complexity of person/environment could best be explored through listening to older people speaking about the fine grain of day-to-day experience encompassing environment in its widest definition.

It followed that the nature and locus of quality in people's lives was more likely to be uncovered through ethnographic exploration with groups and particular cases than through psychometric or statistical measurement. However, in developing the methodology we reconsidered several measures of quality of life in order to compare the experiential categories older people might indicate as significant with those generated by established inventories and scales.

For a largely qualitative study, the data are extensive. We chose three different locations within a 70-mile radius of the Open University headquarters in Milton Keynes: metropolitan/urban (London Borough of Haringey); small town/urban/suburban (Bedford town); and small town/village/semi-rural (Northamptonshire), each with different housing styles and tenures (see Chapter 3). The aim was therefore to reflect the diversity of people and places within the locations.

The late 1990s saw the beginning of greater participation by informants in the research process. Consequently, policymakers and research-funding bodies have welcomed user involvement – sometimes beyond the consultative role and requiring research skills – in the development of services and policies. Certain groups – particularly younger people with disabilities – have experienced this kind of research process as empowering (Peace, 2002). Building on these developments, a decision was taken to begin this research with group discussions to identify themes and categories that older people themselves thought were significant about the places where they lived, both home and community. Nine focus groups were held, comprising three to eight older people. Two groups were assembled specifically for our discussions and the other seven consisted of 'naturally occurring' groups including: two social/luncheon clubs; a mothers' union (Christian) group; a sewing circle; a black oral history group (Haringey); a men's billiards group; and a (Sikh) cultural community group (for which a translator was used) (Bedford). Of the nine groups, four were all-white British and Irish; three were mixed race; one was all-black-Caribbean and one was all Indian. Two of the groups were all male; four were all female; and three were mixed gender. The sessions were led by one or more of the researchers, depending on the size of the group, and they were audiotaped for later content analysis.

Topics raised by the groups included: talking about neighbourhood and community; defining 'my/our place' and belonging; security and

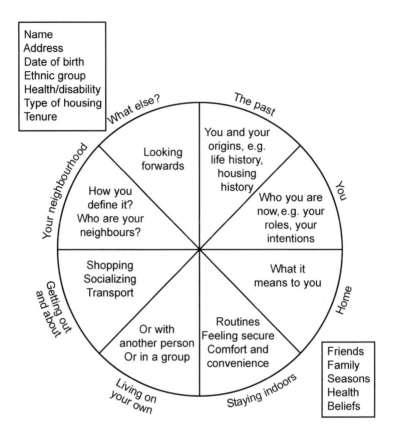

Figure 1.4 Facets of life wheel

insecurity; routines; comfort and convenience; well-being; social engagement and self-agency; 'getting about'; memories. As a result of these discussions a broad interpretation of 'environment' came to underpin our enquiry and taking these leads, a research tool was developed in the form of a rotating circle on a wider board, with eight segments/facets, each containing a topic and prompts – suggested through the group work – for exploration with individuals (see Figure 1.4). A purposive sample of individuals was chosen to cover the housing types common to the varied locations within the three areas. The 54 individual interviews that followed were founded on this new research tool, later called the 'facets of life wheel'.[5]

The eight areas under consideration were:

+ The past (origins; life story; housing history).

+ Self (who are you? now; roles).

+ Home (what it means to you).

+ Staying indoors (routines, comforts, convenience, security).

+ Living arrangements (alone; with another person; in a group).

+ Getting out and about (shopping? socializing? transportation?).

+ Neighbourhood (where is it? what does it mean to you? who are your neighbours?).

+ What else? (including future plans and projects).

As respondents could spin the wheel to read the eight topics and their associated prompts, they could see at a glance the scope of enquiry and control the ordering of discussion by prioritizing the topics that interested them. People were free to elaborate on or add topics or issues that they thought relevant and to ignore whatever did not seem important. It became a prompt for open-ended and recorded discussion. The *facets of life wheel* seemed to enhance people's confidence in collaborating on these themes as they could anticipate the wider context and the ways their particular account might fit. We have already noted how previous approaches to measuring quality of life have tended to use sharply compartmentalized categories that do not allow the best representation of the mutability and continuity of life experience. While based on what can be described as domains of life and living, the *facets of life wheel* seemed, in piloting and in subsequent data collection and analysis, to permit expression of the inter-penetration of social and material aspects of environmental life as this might impact on identity. Moreover, it brings into focus the different and variable intensities that informants can attach to the meanings they ascribe to each of the topics.

While the wheel was the main focus of all of our conversations, to accompany this tool we ensured that we collected basic and supportive data through more structured questions concerning: age, gender, marital status, ethnicity, religion, house type and size, tenure, occupancy, health, financial data, housing satisfaction, housing history,

27

responses to quality-of-life questions from the *Housing Options for Older People* (Heywood et al., 1999), mobility range, accommodation layout and personality characteristics that may influence interaction with the environment. Lists of these areas were included at the sides of the *facets of life wheel* so that respondents understood the range of material being discussed. Consequently, a dossier containing interview transcripts and other data was compiled for each of the respondents – 18 people from each location. Data from transcriptions were subject to content analysis and our aim has been to adopt a grounded theory approach to interpretation (Glaser and Strauss, 1967; Strauss, 1987).

The age of the 54 respondents ranged from 61 to 93 years, with age being defined by individuals seeing themselves as 'an older person' rather than in relation to pensionable age. Sixty-three per cent of the respondents were women and more women than men were interviewed in Northamptonshire. Haringey respondents were the most multi-cultural group of all those who took part in the study: four had been born in the West Indies before coming to Britain in the 1950s, one person had moved from India and two from Ireland while a further respondent, although born in Britain, came from an Italian family. This mixture of nationalities was not seen in the Northamptonshire sample, while in Bedford there were one Anglo-Indian and two Irish respondents.

In terms of housing tenure, those interviewed in Haringey were more likely to be tenants while those in Northamptonshire were more likely to be owner-occupiers. The range of housing covers detached housing to the residential care home. Approaching one-third of our respondents lived in flats, although these were concentrated in Bedford and Haringey. The picture in more rural villages in Northamptonshire tended towards bungalow living (see Chapter 3).

Ethnographic approaches with a relatively small number of respondents, seen intensively over quite long periods, have confirmed the complexity of person/environment interaction and while quality of life issues have remained implicit, findings have justified such methodology. The authors of this research have developed a wide range of methods for data collection: participant observation; in-depth interviewing; taking housing histories; cognitive mapping; collecting photographic records of domestic and special housing interiors; mapping floor plans and furniture arrangements; taking object inventories, and the use of video (Peace, 1977; Peace et al., 1982; Hanson et al., 2001; Holland, 2001). These approaches have accompanied a recognition that people claim that their identities may be influenced by many factors – societal, structural and personal – that impinge on the individual. For example, levels of financial resource, weakening of social networks and incidents of age discrimination need to be seen alongside and interwoven with the personal experiences of an ageing individual who may experience increasing levels of morbidity, degrees of social isolation and sensory loss. The cross-tabulation or multiple regression of these 'factors', 'domains' or 'indicators' no longer seems the most useful approach to exploring the deep complexity of everyday life entailing social and material worlds (see Bornat et al., 2000; Holloway and Jefferson, 2000). In this text, we use the environmental contexts raised by older people to guide the chapters, developing themes that integrate experience with literature.

Structure of the book

Chapters 2 to 7 are based on detailed analysis of material from both focus group work and the 54 in-depth case studies with older people. Chapter 2 offers a temporal perspective on the relationship between older people and the places where they live. Here data on changing housing and households permit an examination of patterns of individuals' accommodation trajectories across the life course, building on Holland (2001). From the respondents' retrospective accounts, we consider the effects of moving and staying put, and of living alone and with other people, on the ways that they approach the possibilities of moving or staying put in later life.

Having considered generational and individual historical material, we move on to focus on everyday living in place. Chapter 3 begins this, considering life beyond the 'garden gate' in the local neighbourhood and community and the geographic/local authority areas of our three study locations in metropolitan, urban and semi-rural areas. Here we discuss how older people locate themselves within community life and do or do not engage with it. Engagement and disengagement are strongly affected by the enabling/disabling environment, access to transport, individual health, financial resources, proximity of family and friends, feelings about security and personal safety and the personal need for engagement.

Moving closer towards the 'home' environment, Chapter 4 takes us to the point of crossing the boundaries to the 'buffer zones' – the inside/outside divide between public and private space. Here we move into that semi-public or semi-private area of the garden, the yard, the communal sitting area and consider the meaning of these different forms of space. For some people appreciating and nurturing nature in urban/rural space is crucial; for others it is a less essential part of their sense of self. Attachment is discussed in relation to territoriality and surveillance and the impact it has on crossing boundaries – physically, visually or aurally.

Chapter 5 seeks to understand the internal life space of the home. Here the focus turns to the routines of daily living and how the home becomes a locus of personal meaning. We describe how older people act on the materialities of the places where they live to maintain a sense of self-in-place that conforms with normative understandings of 'home'. We discuss the notion of the 'life of quality' (Kellaher et al., 2004) that older people strive to develop and sustain and the reader is introduced to the concept of 'option recognition' which the mechanism which we suggest prompts decision making about accommodation and location.

Chapter 6 focuses specifically on specialized housing in the form of sheltered housing and residential care homes. Discussion by respondents who are currently living in these settings and others living in mainstream housing reveal concerns about the extent to which they can facilitate a life of quality in the real sense. The relationship between environment and identity is considered in terms of the facilitation of individual mastery, control, autonomy within dwellings.

Working from the life-course perspective of the individual housing history leads to a rethinking of environmental identity and attachment to place. In Chapter 7, we draw more extensively on six detailed cases to return to the wider understanding of environmental identity that underpins this text. By looking in more detail at these cases, we begin to draw together the threads of time, place and connectivity that we have separated out in the previous chapters.

We end by returning to the question: 'How can the layered environment be drawn on to reflect the complex self in later life?' In Chapter 8, we reflect on the different ways in which the environment is layered and how environmental expression may (or may not) support the engagement of self in different kinds of place and at different times. Consideration is made of commonality in levels of association between environment and identity and associations that are unique to the individual.

To develop these arguments, the essential source of experience rests with the older people with whom we spoke, and we begin our arguments by considering their housing histories.

Notes

1 See *www.enableage.arg.lu.se/about.*

2 See *www.gad.gov.uk/population/1998/engwal/popew98.html.*

3 Discussion of these different datasets and analysis is given in Glaser and Tomassini, 2002.

4 A decision was made not to include in this study nursing home residents or people with severe mental health problem.

5 Five of the respondents took part in making a video entitled 'At Home: place, identity and later life' where they talk about their lives and current living arrangements. The video is available through the authors and may be used for training purposes. Contact: Sheila Peace, Faculty of Health & Social Care, The Open University, Walton Hall, Milton Keynes MK7 6AA.

2

Housing histories

This chapter turns to a consideration of individuals' living environments over time, and the extent to which lifelong experiences of place and of change of place, may have a bearing on how people relate to the places where they live in later life. Our discussion here is based on some general assumptions. First, that everyone's experience of life is unique. Second, that our personal experiences influence but do not define how we deal with personal changes, as well as our attitudes to environment. Third, that where groups of people share some characteristics and live roughly in the same place at the same time, their experience will share certain similarities.

The data collected for the 'Environment and Identity' project included housing histories that are accounts by respondents of the places where they have lived from birth to their present home. Everyone talked about their various 'permanent' homes and some also talked about 'temporary' places where they had lived such as military barracks, hospitals or caravans. Perhaps rather more than is usual in such studies to date, these histories were embedded in other accounts from the respondents about their relationships, health, mobility and in detailed information about present living arrangements and everyday routines. Chapter 1 has described the national picture of the kinds of home where older people currently live in the UK. We wanted to investigate how our respondents' accounts compared with expected patterns of housing moves in response to changes in the life course and with common (and possibly ageist) assumptions about the housing need of older people. We hoped that the relationship between individuals' housing histories and their attachments to home and neighbourhood in later life would emerge from the respondents' accounts of both. This and subsequent chapters describe our analysis of these data.

Chapter 1 also described the design of our research, which empha-sized types of accommodation in three kinds of location. The demographic characteristics of our study sample were in part a con-struct of this design and in part a result of the recruitment techniques we used to find respondents. Consequently, our sample was neither statistically representative (for example of minority ethnic groups; cohorts; wealth) nor comprehensive in its coverage of residential mobility patterns. Nevertheless the amount of detail within the 54 case studies presented us with an unusual opportunity to look at real and situated housing histories in some depth. From these data, and with reference to work previously published by us and by others this chapter investigates how experiences of change and stability in housing affect environment and identity in later life.

Housing histories in 'Environment and Identity'

We invited people to tell us about all the places where they had lived and the data consist of the retrospective accounts produced in response to this invitation. The accounts varied widely in the amount of detail offered – for example, about dates and actual addresses; the apparent ease with which details were remembered; and how the story was told (ordering of the story; number and length of anecdotes, etc.). As might be expected there were very varied experiences of moving house and relocation. Some people had lived in just one or two homes within a tight geographical area; others had experienced international migra-tions and/or moved home very many times throughout their lives. In the following extract, Nullah talks about her present home, to which she had moved in 1959, a couple of years after she was married:

> Well, it was originally a two bedroomed bungalow. But when it was being built, it was a local builder who was building, and he let you say what you wanted. So what we did ... we had stairs put ... it is built as it could be a dorm dormer bungalow, it could have complete dorm dormers each side to make a granny flat or anything upstairs, because it was how the roof was built. So we had stairs put in from the ... second bedroom to make that a little dining room, and windows in the gable end. And so we gradually made a bedroom upstairs for the boys. And then we had a dorm dormer put in on the other side which made a third bedroom, so there is three up there. But recently I have had it altered and had a

shower and a toilet and a little washbasin put up in between the two bedrooms, so that when we have guests you know ... they have got their own. ... And so also we have extended out the back as well, you know, it is quite a big place now I suppose really. (Nullah)

Nullah explained that the original builder of the house had suggested how future adaptations might be incorporated into the design of the house, which seemed to her even then to be a better option than the prospect of having to move as the family grew. This is perhaps an unusually forward-thinking example of the way that people may make adaptations to the places where they live, so that the home physically changes as the household and individuals within it also change. But for most people the story of their living environment involves a series of moves between houses and neighbourhoods. To give a flavour of the kind of histories we encountered in the study, Figure 2.1 represents a brief summary of the housing history of one respondent, Nicola. This woman was aged 76 at the time of the interview and had always lived within a few miles of her birthplace in a small town in North-amptonshire. The figure lists in order the houses she had lived in from birth to the present time, with brief details of her family circumstances. Alongside this information is a description of the kind of accom-modation and who was living in it with her at that time.

One of the key features of Nicola's story is the consistency of living together and family support across and between generations. It gives an example of how the housing histories of individuals intersect and diverge at particular points, as people move into and out of arrange-ments where they share with other people, each of whom will have their own individual housing histories. We can see how decisions about staying put or moving to other accommodation can be profoundly affected by 'significant others'. Describing the housing histories of women, Holland (2001) commented that housing decisions made by and sometimes on behalf of women at different at stages in their lives must be understood in the context of their close social relationships at the time. The 'Environment and Identity' sample, by the time we interviewed the respondents, included 10 still-married people; 39 people who were widow(er)s or divorced/separated; and five people who described themselves as single all their lives or for a very long time. Inevitably, partners strongly influenced each other on housing

	Details	Type of house	Who lived there
First house	1930: Nicola born. Her parents are living with her mother's widowed brother and his two children	Not sure	Nicola, her mum, dad, uncle and two cousins (3 adults, 3 children)
Second house	A few years later uncle remarries so Nicola's parents move. Her father buys a house in the same town: 'It used to have the old fashioned pump thing over the sink, you know, to pour water, they had a pump at the bottom on the entry which went over the sink. Plus we didn't have any bathroom or anything, you know, we had an old fashioned grate'	House – unmodernized terrace	Nicola and her mum and dad (2 adults, 1 child)
	When Nicola is 7, her mother dies		Nicola and her dad (1 adult, 1 child)
Third house	Nicola is aged 11 and her father marries a close neighbour. The new family move to another house	House – 3 bedrooms	Nicola, her dad and her stepmum (2 adults, 1 child)
	Nicola marries in 1948 (aged18) and her husband moves in		Nicola, her dad and stepmum, and her husband (4 adults)
	Two years later her stepmother dies		Nicola, her dad and her husband (3 adults)
	Nicola and her husband continue to live with her father as they have their own three children		Nicola's father (in one bedroom); Nicola, her husband and her daughter (in bedroom two); Nicola's two sons (in bedroom 3) (3 adults, 3 children)
Fourth house	Around the time her daughter was aged 13, the family is able to build a house on local land belonging to Nicola's father, who moves with them (to occupy a ground-floor room).	Bungalow – (purpose-built), 4 bedrooms, 'semi-bungalow'	Nicola and her hus-band; her father; daughter; and 2 sons (3 adults, 3 children)
	After some years her father dies, all the children eventually leave home and, when Nicola is 54, her husband dies: 'So of course the house was too big for me to afford to keep up. So I did an exchange'		(1 adult)
Fifth house	Nicola moves into a smaller house close by	House – 3 bedrooms	(1 adult)
	Eleven years later her oldest son moves back to live with her after the breakdown of his marriage. At the time of interview they have been sharing this home for eight years.		(2 adults)

Figure 2.1 Housing History: Nicola

decisions; but as our respondents talked about how and why they had made changes, they also talked about the influence of their children, parents, siblings and occasionally other family members or friends. Children and other younger family members were often involved in decisions about moving in later life. As people moved into and out of households, they managed adjustments in ways of living alone and with other people, including spatial arrangements, routines and assumptions and expectations about domestic life. We explore some of these issues in more detail later.

Environment, stability and change

A number of our respondents had, in a very literal sense, travelled a long way to find their present homes. For a few people this had involved moving between continents, multiple moves and adjustments to drastic changes in landscape and climate. For others the element of physical travel had been smaller as, like Nicola, they remained close to the home of their birth. Nevertheless the person/environment changes implicit in growing up and growing old within a given time period means that even for people who never move, some physical and symbolic attributes of the home change, and they themselves change over the life course. Consequently, our respondents' experience of home involved a kind of a journey from the childhood home to their present home and presaged their as yet unknown last home.

As it happened, all our respondents had moved house at least once and most had also experienced moving to a different location, for example, to another town or another part of the country. Clark and Dieleman (1996) made a distinction between the kind of house move where one's essential contacts and networks remain intact and those that involve a more drastic reshaping of one's routines:

> [W]hen a move occurs nearby and does not break the web of contacts with friends and work, it can be viewed as a partial displacement ... . Many of the old interactions with friends, family, and even work will not change .... When the move involves a greater separation between the old house and the new house, and there are no, or limited, ties, then the migration is a total displacement migration. (1996, p.41)

Previous experiences of major moves or displacements were recorded in our respondents' histories. We wondered whether these
experiences were reflected in their attitudes to their present living
circumstances. Did they make for a greater sense of security or a lesser
one? To help us think about this particular aspect of environmental
experience, we found it useful to revisit Bourdieu's concept of habitus,
and the sense of one's own (and others') place and role in the world of
experience.

Habitus was conceived as an emphatically fluid construct: 'Being the
product of history, it is an open system of dispositions that is constantly subjected to experiences, and therefore constantly affected by
them in a way that either reinforces or modifies its structures'
(Bourdieu and Wacquant, 1992, p.133). Within given social conditions
the probability is that most people will encounter experiences that tend
to confirm their worldview. However, this is not to say that radical
change cannot take place and Friedmann (2002) has suggested some of
the situations that could bring about fundamental alterations. These
include social mobility, migration, challenge (e.g. by feminist or
fundamentalist ideologies), accelerated change (for example, through
rapid urbanization) and the breakdown of habitus where the social
order has collapsed – either across a whole society or in particular sub-
groups within an otherwise stable society.

As we interpret our respondents' accounts of their various homes
and their movements between them, both family and wider social
contexts (including the locational ones discussed in the next chapter)
continuously mould their take on the world in such a way as to allow
an essential elasticity in modes of living comfortably. Nicola's experience (Figure 2.1) is an illustration of this process. For a few
respondents, disruptive relocations had apparently resulted in radical
changes in outlook. In these cases, one might suggest that the individual's capital resources (Bourdieu, 1986) and personal capacity
(Lawton, 1980) can be detected in the respondent's move forward to a
new environmental balance. Our informant, Bart's experience of
adjusting to an entirely different mode of life following a stroke and
divorce is a very good example of this. Another example is the case of
Harjit, described in detail in Chapter 7. International migration and
traumatic injury each demanded of him particular reconfigurations of
his worldview.

However, for most of our respondents, experiences that tend to confirm one's worldview are reflected in rather more 'evolutionary' changes and in continuities in understandings of home and neighbourhood. Attitudes to and expectations of sharing home space; tenure; age-appropriate behaviour; and, as described in more detail in the next chapter, belonging to particular places – all these factors involve degrees of continuity and change.

In the context of our study, continuity and change are reflected in the narratives within which the respondents present themselves and their housing histories. Laws' (1997) conceptualization of the identity as constantly renegotiated in the context of stereotypes of old age and, in particular, her insistence on the relationship between the discursive identity of individuals and the environments they experience, both hint at the ways in which habitus reflects and affects person/environment interactions. Rubenstein's (1989) conception of the psychosocial processes linking person to place and Rubenstein and Parmelee's later (1992) description of the time and space elements of personal attachment – transforming *space* into *place* – inform our analysis of the respondents' reflections on environments of meaning.

The average age of the respondents in 'Environment and Identity' was 80 years (range 61 to 93). In considering their housing histories, it is important to retain a sense of the socio-historic context of these lives. Their personal housing choices and interpretations have been influenced to a greater or lesser degree by the large-scale events and trends of the 20th century, including war; migration patterns; increasing affluence; education; technological change; and changing attitudes within and between cohorts, to name but some. Historic changes in the availability and affordability of housing during this period also have a bearing on individual and family decisions at particular points and Holland (2001) has discussed the differential effects on the housing experience of people in different cohorts within this generation.

Historic context also affects attitudes and helps to mould habitus. When people of this generation talk about the homes they lived in as children and young adults, it is not uncommon for them to talk about the domestic standards of their parents and grandparents (or employers in the case of domestic or military service) in influencing their own attitudes. For example, Beatrice said:

I mean I know we shouldn't look back, but erm for instance when I make my bed in the morning, the lady that I was companion to in London, she was very strict with everything and if her pillows didn't have the crease down the centre, or her sheets wasn't the dead centre, when she went to bed she used to have me out of my bed and I had to strip it all and do it again.

[*Interviewer*: Now do you still keep those standards yourself?]

Yes. That crease must still be in my sheet, and ... my husband used to get so cross with me. Because his mother was the same more or less, you know she was in private service. (Beatrice)

Yet ideas and attitudes arising within one generation can permeate broader society in such a way as to change the attitudes of earlier or later generations – particularly where the new approaches or ideas are attractive. Riggs and Turner (2000) suggested that, depending on events, older generations may become highly influenced by the social behaviours of younger ones. Respondents in 'Environment and Identity' had both influenced, and been influenced by, younger generations in their own family, and by changing social attitudes generally. It would be a mistake to assume that the transfer of knowledge is a one-way affair.

For Mannheim (1997), a key agent of social change was the cohort. For him, generation, like class, is a category that exists whether or not its members are aware of it. The commonality of experience of historic events, or in his terms the 'stratification of experience' is a dynamic process, encapsulating a notion of 'generation units' or groups of people within the same generation who may have held oppositional attitudes to the same events. (Klatch, 1999, for example has described ideological and gender differences within the '60s' generation'). Significantly for the purposes of this discussion, Mannheim suggests that the 'viewpoint' of older generations is unlikely to match well the experience of younger generations, especially in times of accelerated change. Arguably then, the continuous spoken and unspoken dialogues between cohorts and generations are integral to the continuous revision of habitus and what is taken by older people as confirmatory of their worldview and what challenges it. Within the 'Environment and Identity' housing histories, this process can be seen in attitudes to multigenerational living, tenure and place rootedness; all of which are discussed in more detail later in this chapter and in Chapter 3.

The housing 'journey'

While some households choose not to move or are not able to do so, the housing histories of families have most commonly been described as histories of mobility. The life course/housing connection is most obvious when people move house in response to life events such as marriage, childbirth or retirement. Not surprisingly, much of the early literature on housing histories was based on studies of residential mobility. Rossi (1955) investigated household residential mobility in Philadelphia and found that housing requirements were strongly linked to lifecycle phase. He stated that short-distance moves in particular could be explained as efforts to satisfy 'needs' brought about by life-cycle changes.

Subsequent writers have worked with the notion of life course rather than the more deterministic lifecycle, some using a biographical approach. Clark and Dieleman (1996) identified this life-course approach to residential mobility as originating in sociological and psychological lifecycle stages and/or categorizations, with an emphasis on linear progression through an imagined traditional lifecycle as 'new couples' move on through family formation to old age and probably to living alone. Moving has been studied in the context of employment, changing household size, increasing affluence and market change; and models of choice and constraint have been employed to expand on notions of rational behaviour in housing acquisition (see Holland, 2001, Chapter 3).

From these studies, some broad trends in housing mobility were identified. For example, there was some evidence from empirical studies that working-class families were likely to be less mobile than middle-class families (Clapham et al., 1993). Opportunities to move may be restricted within particular housing markets and, as we have implied, households may have many factors to take into account (such as work, local connections and affordability) in addition to the suitability of their housing when deciding whether or not to move. Mobility studies have also looked at events that might predispose households to move 'down' at later stages in the lifecycle; for example when children leave home, when people retire from work and after becoming widowed; and at the migration of older people from Britain. For example Warnes (1991) and King et al. (2000) have looked at

British migration in later life to the Mediterranean area, where migrants have tended to be more affluent (and certainly none of our respondents realistically expected to make such a move).

Large-scale migration studies have thus dealt with broad social movements and often with theoretical lives. Yet real-life families and households are more elastic than the buildings that house them. Looking in detail at the specific housing histories of individuals, as we have done in this study, tends to produce more finely grained data within which patterns may be discerned in the complexity of people's actual lives.

The analysis we offer here is at this level: local, specific and indicative, but not presented as a definitive account of mobility at the national scale. At the broadest level, it was possible to see patterns of similarity within the uniqueness of the respondents' housing histories based on the frequency and timing of moves.

Patterns in respondents' housing histories

Relocation

Migrants

Some respondents had moved house several times and by the time we interviewed them had settled in a place far from their place of birth. This group included people who had migrated to Britain at some point, most of them in early adulthood to take up work or further education. Common elements in the housing narratives of this group of people included the effects on their younger selves of a new physical and social environment; the process of getting settled to some degree in the new environment; and the tensions, once they had become settled in their new homes, in their sense of belonging. This process is discussed in more detail in Chapter 7, in the case of Harjit.

Movers

Another subgroup of people had relocated several times. Some had been born and raised in the UK, but had lived abroad for some time before returning to Britain. Others had relocated, often several times, but always within the UK. This group included some people who had lived elsewhere at various stages, but had for one reason or another moved back fairly close to the place where they had lived as children.

Locals

While all the respondents in our sample happened to have moved at least once in their lives, another subgroup had moved house very infrequently as adults and had also tended to stay 'local' thus more or less avoiding disruptive relocations and maintaining some continuity with the significant places in their lives.

Within these patterns of movements between *locations*, the housing histories also showed different patterns of moves between different *kinds* and *tenures* of accommodation including houses and flats of various sizes and accommodation that was shared or not shared and in good or poor condition. In Chapter 3, we go on to consider the importance of location and in Chapter 5, we go into more detail about the physicality of current homes and their effect on the identity and well-being of the respondents in later life. Figure 2.2 shows the tenure range within the 'Environment and Identity' respondents at the time of interview; Figure 2.3 shows the different types of housing that they lived in.

Tenure

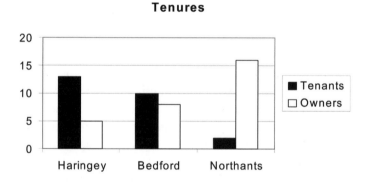

Figure 2.2 Tenure range in the study

Following the Thatcherite reversal of post-war council housing development, the late 1980s produced a certain amount of academic debate about the significance of housing tenure. Saunders and Williams (1988), for example, argued that because the home is simultaneously a social and physical location it potentially offers some people a source of 'ontological security': a sense of niche and belonging which reflects persistence in place and time: *'Cars and television sets belong to people, but it is people themselves who feel that they "belong" at home'* (Saunders and Williams, 1988, p.87). Saunders later (1990) described the economic benefits of home ownership, which allows the accumulation and transmission of wealth; and its enhancement of autonomy by reinforcing attitudes of independence. But he also suggested that ownership *of itself* conferred both actual and emotional security. He suggested that ownership or non-ownership was therefore a major factor in determining how people felt about their homes.

However, 'belonging at home' might not mean the same thing as having a home belong to you: a person could feel either, both or neither. Hamnett (1991), Watt (1993) and others disputed the Saunders and Williams' interpretation, while accepting the significance of tenure as an important issue and Gurney (1999) described the normalizing discourse that is now embedded in the discussion of home ownership. This suggested a new form of social exclusion that might be experienced by those who continue to rent their homes.

As we describe in Chapter 3, there were differences between our three study areas both in the tenure patterns of the local populations and in the tenure of our respondents in those areas. Although many other respondents had lived in rented accommodation at earlier points in their lives, most of them were currently living in houses that they owned (although a few of the respondents had moved out of ownership back into renting or into a residential care home). Twenty-nine of our respondents were living at the time we interviewed them in houses that they owned, and most of these were owned outright. Another 19 were renting their accommodation and six were living in residential care homes as licensees. Most of our respondents who were currently renting were living in sheltered housing or housing that was purpose built for older people (previously referred to as 'Part One' accommodation).

As our respondents tactically maintained a life of quality, being able to hold onto their own homes was a clear priority and one that might be expected. While for some of our respondents the actual house was crucial, for others the neighbourhood or the social and family positioning of the home was more critical. Furthermore, their present tenure has to be seen in the context of their whole-life housing history and in the account of how they moved from where they started in life to where they are now and hoped to be in the future. We are therefore reading tenure as part of the layered environment that the respondents constantly interpreted and negotiated. They tended to reflect norma-tive expectations that ownership (outright) would provide more security in terms of being able to stay put, but perhaps be more of a problem in terms of maintenance and costs. People who had not been owner-occupiers were more likely either to have moved into sheltered accommodation or to consider it as a future possibility.

Housing types

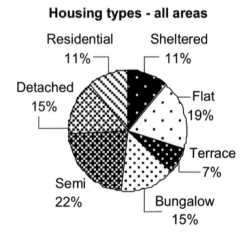

Housing types - all areas

Figure 2.3 Housing types in the study

One of the key features of this study was the diversity of types of accommodation (Figure 2.3). We go on, in Chapter 5, to say more about the effects of different forms on accommodation on the well-being of the respondents, but here we concentrate on the paths that brought them to be living in their present accommodation.

While a few of our respondents had lived in many different kinds of accommodation and in different places, most had at least had some experience of houses or flats other than where they lived now; and it was these experiences that seemed to colour their views of their present accommodation rather than the type and size of the accommodation itself. For example Belinda living alone in a three-bedroomed house with a large garden did not find it particularly large relative to her previous home and her current lifestyle; while Betty, after a lifetime of domestic work was very satisfied with the relatively modest space of a flat in a sheltered housing scheme.

Given that all of our respondents who were not living in residential care homes were to a greater or lesser degree content with physical aspects of their current accommodation, regardless of its size and tenure, we wanted to consider also their own perceptions of the relative status of their home. Here again, people could position both their homes and their neighbourhoods relative to others – for example some people compared their own modest homes to those of their more affluent children – but it was their subjective assessment of having themselves moved 'up' or 'down' in life that was important and their housing was part of this assessment.

Moving 'up' (and 'down') in life

One group of respondents considered themselves, on balance, to have 'moved up' in relation to the house(s) where they had started out as children, or lived for most of their adult lives. They included Norman who had inherited a significant family home; and Belinda who felt she had moved into a neighbourhood that suited her much better. It included people who had moved in mid-life from renting to buying their home; and people who had 'downsized' but felt that their smaller accommodation was superior (for example, in location or tenure) to where they had lived before.

In contrast, another group of respondents implied that they had 'moved down' relative to earlier homes and especially in comparison to childhood homes. Examples here are Bob who moved into sheltered housing to give his house to his son's family; Bart who was forced to move into a council rented flat following divorce and disability; and all but one of the people now living in residential care homes.

A third group of respondents felt that the status of their homes had remained more or less the same. This included people who had stayed put or moved to a similar type or standard of accommodation – often in the same or a similar kind of location. However, it must be said that some of these had also gained financially in real terms through the increased value of their house.

The final group had a more complex pattern. For example Betty, after a relatively wealthy childhood in a large house, had been a resident housekeeper for many years before retiring to a council flat. While she had been used to living for most of her life in more affluent surroundings, her present sheltered flat was all her own and also an improvement on the council flat.

By inviting us into their homes for the interviews, respondents were demonstrating some confidence in the status of their homes at least in terms of their being presentable to strangers. People living in places that they consider to be unpresentable or completely unsuited to their own status are probably less likely to volunteer to take part in this kind of in-depth probing. Further research is needed into the effects of changing environmental status on the identity of people who feel marginalized in these terms.

The idea of moving (again) in later life

We would argue that the dialectic between autonomy and security (Lawton, 1980) is played out across housing histories as people negotiate location, tenure and types of accommodation; and that it comes particularly into focus when people consider the pros and cons of moving in later life. The balancing of the potential and probable benefits and costs of specific alternatives (including the status quo) becomes more important to maintaining independence and self-confidence.

We asked all the respondents whether they had thought about moving on from their present home and whether they thought it was likely that they would move in the foreseeable future. A few people had moved comparatively recently and we asked how they had decided to move and whether they were happy with the move. Another group had decided that they would probably need to move, either in the short or longer term. More people had seriously thought about the possibility of moving from their present home but for various reasons had decided against it, at least for the present. The final group had either not thought seriously about moving or had decided not to give it too much thought.

The prospect of moving later in life is especially difficult when people are living alone or in poor health. The amount of disruption involved, quite apart from the organization and costs of the move itself, are serious considerations that may well outweigh the possible benefits of a prospective new home over the present one. In addition, the move itself may be seen as a negative action compared to other, more positively regarded house moves (such as to accommodate children, or a new job; or to move into a bigger, better house) – for example. Steinfeld (1981) remarked on this in relation to moving into sheltered housing. Nevertheless, some of the respondents had moved or were seriously thinking about it. The person who had moved most recently was Beryl, who following the recent death of her husband, had felt unable to cope alone. Determined not to live with her children, she had been helped by them to move into a residential care home close to a daughter's home, but far away from her friends and her previous home. In doing so she had also moved from owning her own home to becoming a licensee. Beryl clearly missed her old home and her husband, but felt that in her present state of health she had made the right decision. Yet this was the very radical change of status that many of the respondents were most anxious to avoid and in Chapter 6 we go on to consider why.

Some of our respondents said that they had been thinking about moving, either to sheltered housing or another place. For some people such a move was little more that a possible event at some unspecified future time; others regarded it more as a probability – but when the time and accommodation was right for them. While not ruling out their futures in age-specific homes, our respondents, like those of many other studies, were inclined to put off both the decision and the move, in spite of the gentle encouragement of their families:

> So she said 'why don't you put in for one of the little bungalows or flats?' and I said 'I don't want one yet' and she said 'but at least you have got your name down' and I said 'I don't want to move there yet, I like my life in Rushden, all my friends are here you know'. I said 'perhaps in another 10 years time I might think about it'. You know, and she said 'if you sold your house you could have a granny flat' and I said 'No'. (Nicola, aged 76)

Most of the respondents thought that they would think more seriously about moving if and when their health and strength started to fail them. But, as with other studies of this kind, a good number said that they had no intention of moving unless 'carried out'. This was particularly true of respondents who were very attached to the actual house in which they had lived for a long time and which had become a strong support to their sense of identity. We give a particular example of this kind of attachment in Chapter 7.

For most of our respondents, moving or not moving was bound up with uncertainty about their future selves. Any of us may find our plans or aspirations thwarted by circumstances, but the respondents were dealing with the additional factor, expressed (usually) or not, that increasing age would increase the likelihood that their present living arrangements would have to change and that they would have to face death. Whether thinking positively or negatively about moving again or indeed choosing to ignore the possibility, respondents were aware that any further move might well be the last and this appeared to be a more daunting thought than that of remaining where they were. In spite of or perhaps because of these uncertainties, respondents tended to value their present living arrangements whatever they were, appreciating those aspects of home that supported their sense of well-being and self-determination and allowed them to live the life of quality that they did not want to lose. For most of our respondents this included a sense of being in the right location or neighbourhood. The respondents' strategies for maintaining comfortable and fulfilling living arrangements therefore had a quality of conditionality to them, combining resilience with hope and a determination to make the best of things that might be beyond their own control.

A further strong theme within the housing histories concerned the issue of living arrangements, specifically alone or with other people, at different periods in life and particularly with increasing age.

Living arrangements: living as 'family' and as 'alone'

I have the three children, and my father was getting on in years, 86 you see, and erm ... we wanted a bigger place, so he had some ground and he turned that over to me and we had a bungalow built, well semi-bungalow, four bedroomed, along there. But ... we had a room for him downstairs, because ... we only got three bedrooms in [previous house] you see, and I had got two boys and a girl, and the girl had to sleep in my room until she was about 13, until we moved. My husband had made a bathroom because he was a decorator in business, in that house, modernized it. So of course we sold that and had a room downstairs for dad. And I looked after him until he was 89, and then ... the children grew up, left home, and got married. And then unfortunately my husband died at 63, I was 54. So of course the house was too big for me to afford to keep up. So I did an exchange, a builder had got this house and he wanted one down there, so I did an exchange. And then my eldest son, his marriage fell apart so he came back here to live with me, which he does now. (Nicola)

Here Nicola, whose housing history we outlined in tabular form at the beginning of this chapter, describes in her own words the events prompting her last two house moves. Hers was a common enough experience of the deals and compromises that families make to live together comfortably within the available accommodation. (We are using the shorthand phrase 'families' here, primarily meaning nuclear and extended groups of relatives, but also to include significant 'family-like' others.) In Nicola's three-bedroomed house (the third house in Table 2.1) there was a problem of overcrowding – certainly within standard definitions of occupancy at the time. In this case, her father happened to own some land and her husband was a builder, so as family their favoured solution was to construct a larger house with a room on ground-floor level for the older man. One might speculate that in other circumstances, her father might have gone into residential care or perhaps have been supported to remain in his own house. In time Nicola's children had moved on, her father and husband had died. She decided to move to accommodation that would suit her, living alone, as an older women. But before long her son was sharing the house with her, as their housing histories crossed again.

Nicola's description of her moves from house to house does clearly demonstrate some of the concerns of relocation studies – moving in response to household expansion and contraction; rational use of markets; choice within constraints. And for Nicola there was also need to deal with the unexpected – the death of her husband; the return of her married son; and with personal and social expectations – to care and to share and to maintain a continuity of family life. Furthermore, the homes were not just about her, being elements in the housing histories of the other people in the story. In the three houses mentioned in the last quotation, Nicola's homes were at one and the same time the childhood homes of her children; a house her husband modernized and another he built; her father's final home; and a refuge for her son after the break-up of his marriage. So each house contained people at different stages in their life course and with different priorities and expectations, and it is these interactions that make housing histories so much more complex than simple patterns of household moves can indicate.

The 'Environment and Identity' data show many examples of housing compromises as people seek to maintain essential relationships. For example, moves to take up a new job (usually by the male partner in couples) included calculations about the effects of taking a particular job on the rest of the household. Sometimes people had decided not to take jobs rather than leave places that were important to them. In a few cases, couples had split up after moving, when one partner decided they really wanted to move back to a place where they felt they belonged. Sometimes individuals took on a long commute to work to allow the rest of the family to stay put. Decisions about who would and who would not be part of a particular household showed similar compromises, with the intergenerational and by-marriage obligations of one person in a household being mediated by others in that household (and also, in some cases, by non-resident family members).

The result was that family considerations, in addition to extending options (for example, the possibility of moving back in with mother) could also restrict the options available to individuals, if they wanted to keep in step with the rest of the family. In the case of couples making decisions, one might say that their options were as likely to be halved as doubled. Bernard and Brian for example, both said that they would have preferred to move were it not for the opinions of their wives.

Forty-four of the respondents were living alone at the time of interview. Of these, 39 people had previously been married with children. Four people had never been married and most had lived alone for many years. In addition, many respondents had lived alone during earlier periods of their lives and a few said they had thought about a possible future of living alone. Needless to say, experiences varied considerably, as did the degree to which living alone was a preference rather than a necessity. Among those living alone at the time of interview, independence was a significant rationale. The notion of independence has been described as including elements of privacy and self-determination, competence and status (WHO, 2000) and, in the case of older people, it is an essential part of the rhetoric of satisfactory housing. When they talked about living alone, our respondents sometimes talked about the benefits of being able to do what they liked when they liked and not having to be answerable to anyone else or having to fit into their routines. However, when directly questioned whether or not they had sufficient human company, people who were now living alone were the most likely to say that sometimes they were lonely. Most accepted the ambiguities of living alone in preference to the available alternatives; nevertheless there were many regrets about the loss of a partner.

In Chapter 7, we describe in detail the experience of one of the respondents who lived alone, but very much with the presence of her late husband in her thoughts and in her relationship with the house and neighbourhood. Other women and men in the study described similar experiences, certainly in the first years following the death of a spouse and in some cases for many years afterwards. For some, the 'shadow' spouse still figured in their thinking and feelings about the home and contents. For example, in the course of his recorded interview, Harry mentioned his wife, who had been deceased for four years, 37 times in two hours.

This evident need to keep something of the spouse alive by having a consideration for their preferences while alive, was stronger in the narratives of some rather than others among the widowed respondents and some people did feel able to made changes because they no longer had to be constrained by their partner. This tendency to bear in mind another (absent) person's needs is not exclusive to widowed people and the small number of single people in our sample had strong ties to other members of their family such as cousins or nephews. Just as older people may, according to Rowles (1978), have reference to 'fantasy' places that are significant within their own world of meaning, so we would argue that the memory or imagining of significant other people allows them to continue an essential family life while living alone. In addition to requiring space for visitors, including bedroom space, many of our respondents used space in their own homes temporarily or permanently for the belongings of other people, as a very practical way of maintaining relationships. It is one of the shortcomings of much housing provision for older people that this need for family life is not taken into account.

In living alone, most of our respondents took care to avoid, as far as possible, being lonely. In many cases, especially among the women, widowhood had been their first real taste of living alone and many of them described how older relatives in their own birth families had been looked after to avoid loneliness. For example, Bertha described an arrangement that was possibly more common when she was young than it is now, although it still happens in some situations. Children could be looked on both as assets in terms of company and help around the house and liabilities in terms of financial support and nurturing. On this basis they might be 'shared' within extended families. One of eight children of an Irish family, Bertha lived as a girl for seven years with her step-grandmother in Scotland. *'Well, she wanted me to you know .... She begged my mum and dad. And of course they had a big family, there was a lot of them. You can spare one, I was the one.'* A consciousness of the vulnerability of older relatives to loneliness was also shown in the histories of several other respondents who had lived with their grandparents, or had later shared a home with their own ageing parents. Nevertheless the 20th-century dominance of the ideal of independence had so permeated approaches to old age that, in common with respondents in many other studies (Toffaleti, 1997; Clark et al., 1998; Heywood et al., 1999), most of our respondents regarded independence, even if it entailed some loneliness, as desirable and in many ways morally superior to 'being a burden' on their family and this was a key element in the acceptability of living alone in later life.

If we consider the socio-historical context for this group and the ways in which developments in housing provision and household formation may well have been reflected within intergenerational 'dialogues' on appropriate or optimal behaviour, the housing histories themselves offer some kind of an explanation. Most of our respondents, like the vast majority of people in the 1920s and 1930s, were born into families that lived in private rented accommodation. For many people this accommodation was substandard by today's definitions and often it was shared with extended family. Like many people during this period, several respondents had left formal education at around 14 years; others later; but in almost all cases where possible they continued to live in their parents' or guardians' homes until they married or went into military or domestic service or nursing.

Understandably accounts vary on the ease or difficulty of these arrangements but there was usually a clear presumption of the authority of the parent generation. However, following the social dislocations of World War Two and post-war economic material and social reconstruction, it became much more viable for young adults to find and maintain homes of their own and many of the respondents saw significant improvements in their own housing situations. Respondents in our study, as in many others, often told us with pride about the subsequent achievements of their children and grandchildren – getting degrees; securing good jobs, sometimes abroad; buying their own houses. Becoming, in fact, independent of them, at least in material ways. This appeared to draw general social approval. Like their own parents, our respondents wanted to be good parents, but for many their understanding of what this meant had changed. 'Not being a burden' now appeared to be more important than having an accepted role in giving direction and guidance to the next generation. For example, Bernard was adamant that he did not want to go into an age-specific 'little box', but when asked about the possibility of living with his children he responded:

[Gasps] Even worse! Even worse, I couldn't do it, no way, no way would I inflict myself on my children. My wife is of the same mind, our children have both said if anything happens to one or the other, the one that is left will come and stay with us. No. No. If it is a choice with living with my daughter and living in a little box, I think I would go for living in the little box. (Bernard)

Of course, this pattern did not apply to all our respondents, but these experiences of changing expectations about intergenerational living appeared common enough to indicate a partial explanation for the strength of the current emphasis by many older people on living independently. Whether such attitudes will persist in future generations of older people will depend to a large extent on the housing histories currently being lived in a still-changing housing market.

Conclusion

The respondents in this study generously gave us their housing histories, each very different from the next, yet bearing the similarities that we have begun to describe in this chapter. Their histories underpinned their current housing circumstances and status and their attitudes to both of these. The histories mattered both because past housing opportunities had a material influence on the housing that was realistically available to individuals now and because they formed an essential part of the context within which respondents evaluated their current circumstances. This is not to say that previous experiences determined current (or future) housing outcomes and clearly the influence of past homes was felt more strongly by some than by others. Movements earlier in life that had resulted in social dislocation, whether or not experienced at the time as traumatic, had, by the time we interviewed the respondents, become part of the narrative of self, but without, any longer, strongly expressed potency in everyday life. In particular, people with a history of relocation tended to interpret this as a sign of resilience. Yet as we shall see in subsequent chapters neither this kind of experience, nor one of long-term residence and stability, could necessarily protect respondents against the prospect of making a final disruptive move into residential care.

What we are discussing throughout this book is the edited accounts of their lives that the respondents gave to us and that we subsequently interpreted. We have not been with them on their journey through various homes and neighbourhoods. We were, however, present at their current locations (and the site for many of most of their lives) and in the next chapter we turn to the particularities of place.

3
Location, location, location

As we discussed in Chapter 2, respondents in the 'Environment and Identity' study told us about their various experiences of relocation and migration and of continuity and change in the places where they had lived. In this chapter, we look in more detail at the significance of location in their everyday lives as older people. We begin the chapter by considering conceptual understandings of place and of what it is that fosters the sense of attachment to place. Then we introduce in more detail the three study locations (Bedford, Haringey and North-amptonshire) before considering some of the findings from focus group sessions and individual interviews.

A sense of place

We believe that where an older person lives is an essential element in their quality of life and not merely a 'setting' within which the life is lived. Laws (1997) and Dixon and Durrheim (2000) are among the many geographers and environmental psychologists who subscribe to the interactivity of persona and place: place being seen as important in allowing people to create and sustain a sense of self. People may want and need to be in different kinds of place at different periods in their lives. In an ideal world, each of them would be 'the right place' at 'the right time'. But the appropriateness of particular places for particular people is bound up with complexities of continuity and change, so that people can find themselves to be 'out of place' and experiencing a diminished quality of life.

What do we mean by 'a sense of place'? It is a concept that has been

discussed in many disciplines – social science and sociology, anthropology, environmental psychology, geography and architecture among
them. It is clear that while many authors attest that 'sense of place' exists
and is vitally important both to individuals and societies, no single
definition of sense of place has emerged from these various approaches.
Nevertheless there are certain commonalities in what have been regarded as key aspects to understanding how people interact with the places
where they live and work. These themes have included the following:

Knowledge of place

To have a sense of place it is necessary to know it in some way.
Arguably, the more intimately one knows a place, the better one's sense
of it, for better or worse. Place knowledge is seen as related both to
memory and to interpretation and to embrace legends, myths and the
'spirit of place'. Experience and stories help a place to become legible to
the person and in this process knowing the name (or naming) of the
place plays an important part; so too does a physical knowledge
through bodily experience. Narratives of individual and group
experience can help to define and explain places and embed the
received cultural understandings of them.

Connection through identity

Place therefore has biographical relevance. People generally forge
attachments to places as part of their everyday lives and a sense of real
connectedness can be made at almost any stage of life and to more than
one significant place. Yet individuals may also form attachments to
places by virtue of the collective identity or history of groups with
which they closely identify (such as religious or cultural groups). Both
individual and collective responses to such culturally significant places
can include emotional and spiritual attachments to them in people
who personally know them very little or not at all. But while a person
might claim a strong attachment to such a place, it could be argued
that lack of personal knowledge and familiarity produces a 'real'
attachment to a place that is 'imagined'.

Consequences of loss of place

Because people live always in time and place, and because of their
intimate connections with specific places, loss of place is seen as a

serious disadvantage. Homelessness and rootlessness are related to social alienation and exclusion and to losing the sense of one's past (and therefore, arguably, one's future). This argument has been applied both to individuals and to displaced groups, where loss of place may also imply the loss of cultural heritage and community cohesion.

Mechanisms of attachment

Place attachment, an outcome of knowledge and connection and, we would argue, an aspect of identity, has been defined as an affective bond between people and place or setting (Tuan, 1974). The inter-disciplinary nature of interest in person/place relationships is evident in the range of analytical frameworks that have been used to describe how people form and maintain attachments to places. These have included interpretive, interactionist, constructionist and social construction behaviours, experiential cultural beliefs and behaviours (Low, 1992; Milligan, 1998). As we will discuss later in this chapter, it is essential to the quality of life of older people that they are able to actively maintain their connections to the places where they live.

A suitable place for old age?

Is there then such a thing as 'a suitable place' in which to grow old? Wahl, in discussing the early role of environmental gerontology within the discipline noted 'the long prevailing tendency in gerontology to assign priority to the person and to neglect the physical and spatial circumstances that provide an important contextual element for aging' (Wahl, 2003, p.6). By the 1970s the role of living environments was increasingly being considered, but largely within contexts of indoor environments, especially age-specific settings such as residential facilities. This accompanied a tendency to understand the older person as 'vulnerable' to environment and as rather passive in the face of environmental challenges. Later developments in environmental gerontology (see Chapter 1) and in understandings of the ageing process have moved to positions that emphasize the aspirations of most older people to remain in their own homes and neighbourhoods for as long as possible and acknowledge the proactivity of older people as they engage with their environments. As we have shown in the previous chapter, most of our respondents had a conditional plan to stay put if possible and we will go on in later chapters to describe their engagements with environment to enable them to achieve a life of an acceptable quality in the place where they preferred to be.

The fact is that individual older people are complex social beings for whom sense of place is intrinsic to ontological security and who, for the most part, actively pursue living circumstances that promote a life of quality in their own terms. The diversity of older people and the acknowledgement by policymakers of the need for choice in housing (ODPM, 2001) already indicate that there are problems with attempting to define 'a suitable place' for old age in general, as distinct from a place that might be suitable for a particular older person. In the 'Environment and Identity' study we wanted to consider a contemporary representation of what factors allow older people to feel that they are in their own 'right place'. In subsequent chapters, we go into detail about our findings in relation to individual homes and types of accommodation. In this chapter, we explore the significance of the locations of those homes, beginning with a description of each of our three study locations. We then go on to discuss what the respondents in both the focus groups and the individual interviews told us about their relationships with these (and other) locations. In essence what we are considering here are aspects of living in urban and rural locations and the implications of forming and maintaining attachments to these places.

The three study areas

The study sites in 'Environment and Identity: a cross-setting study' were selected to include elements of different levels of urbanization as part of our cross-section of accommodation types. In Haringey, a borough within the international city of London, we found that people might identify with the different parts of Haringey or with London in general as much as with the borough itself. In Bedford, we had a town with strong historic identity and a well-established place within its county and the wider area. Northamptonshire, by way of contrast, was a diverse county with a population dispersed between Northampton itself, the rural areas, and a collection of smaller towns. It had complex administrative arrangements and diverse and distinct communities across the county – so that, for example, East Northamptonshire, with

Table 3.1 Comparative population data

2001	England	Haringey	Bedford	Northamptonshire			
				South	East	Kettering	Wellingborough
Population	49,138,831	216,507	147,911	79,293	76,550	81,844	72,519
Average age	38.6	34.1	37.8	38.6	38.5	38.7	38.6
One-person households	30.0	35.9	28.0	23.4	25.8	27.9	28.2
Pensioners living alone	14.4	10.3	13.1	12.1	12.4	13.3	13.6
Other all-pensioner households	9.4	3.8	9.2	9.3	9.8	9.7	9.2
% white	90.9	65.6	87.0	98.4	98.3	96.7	90.8
% Christian	71.8	50.1	68.8	77.8	73.3	71.6	68.2

Source: www.statistics.gov.uk/about/census

no obvious core, was described as having a lack of geographical cohesion that 'challenges our community identity' (ENCC, 2003). The comparative population statistics (2001 census) for the three study areas are given in Table 3.1.

House prices in both Bedford and Northamptonshire tended on average to be lower than the national average and in the southeast, but higher than in the East Midlands.

Some respondents in these areas were aware of pressures on house prices and availability, especially for younger people in their communities:

> We are getting a lot of people coming in now, probably from the south who have sold properties at high prices, and they are coming in and prepared to pay high prices here. Which of course doesn't help ... the normal people here, you know the residents here because it is quite a low paid area really. But then there is a lot of people in higher paid jobs, it is difficult to know how to strike the balance. (Nullah)

Compared to both Bedford and Northamptonshire, house prices in Haringey were very high. Table 3.2 shows the comparative tenure patterns of the local authority areas in 2001. We have described the tenure breakdown of the people we interviewed in Chapter 2 (page 42); most of our Haringey respondents rented while most of the Northamptonshire residents were owner-occupiers.

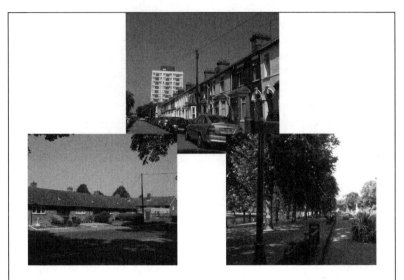

Bedford

The town of Bedford contains most of the population of the present administrative borough of Bedford, claimed as the second oldest English borough (chartered 1166). It has been described as having a 'prosperous hinterland' (*BBC News*, 2003), with the town's population[1] weighted towards professional, managerial and skilled employment. At the 2001 census, 87% of Bedford's residents were white and 72% of its households were owner-occupiers. Our research included people living in the older established town centre areas of Bedford and in areas of later council housing and private developments on the edge of the town. In the second phase of the research we interviewed eight men and ten women in Bedford, aged from 63 to 93 years. Ten of these respondents were tenants and eight were owner-occupiers. Fourteen people lived alone, three with a partner and one with an adult child. Four people had seriously limiting physical disabilities and two had serious medical conditions.

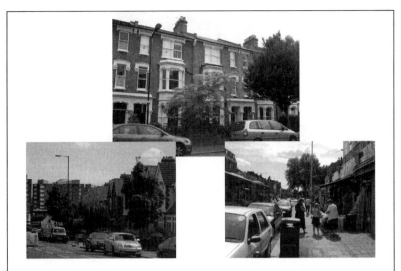

Haringey

Haringey is an outer London borough, described as having 'inner London challenges' (LBH, 2003). It was established in 1964 by the amalgamation of the former boroughs of Hornsey, Wood Green and Tottenham. At the 2001 census, there was a population of 216,510 people within 11.5 sq. miles (73.2 per hectare), skewed toward people aged 20 to 40 years – just 13% of the population were aged over 60 years compared to the UK average of around 20%. Haringey is a multicultural borough. Almost 66% of Haringey residents registered as white. Eighteen per cent of people identified themselves as black-Caribbean or black-African by origin – these being the two largest minority ethnic groups in the borough. The housing stock in Haringey is varied, with a large number of sheltered housing units. The housing and socioeconomic profile of the borough has given rise to a fairly recognizable difference between the Tottenham area and the generally more affluent areas of Hornsey and Wood Green. Our research was conducted in all parts of the borough and we interviewed seven men and eleven women, aged from 66 to 88 years. Three people had serious limiting physical disabilities. Thirteen respondents were tenants and five were owner-occupiers. Seventeen people lived alone and one with a partner.

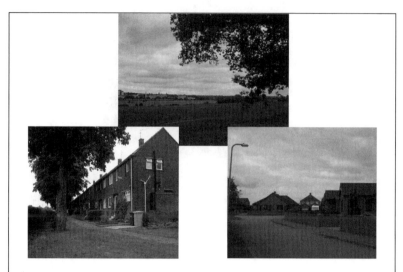

Northamptonshire
The region covered by Northamptonshire County Council includes seven district and borough councils.[2] Our research was conducted primarily in Kettering, Wellingborough and South and East Northamptonshire. The size of settlements included in our research ranged from Kettering (population 47,000), Rushden (24,000) Burton Latimer (7000) and Towcester (7000), to Rushton (400).[3] Overall, these towns and villages had much less ethnic diversity (90–98% white origin) than the other two locations. On average, around 20% of the populations were aged over 60 and there was a high rate (72–79%) of owner-occupation (Table 3.2). We interviewed five men and 13 women, aged from 72 to 82. Thirteen people lived alone and five with a partner; two people had seriously limiting physical disabilities and two had seriously limiting mental health problems. Two people were tenants and 16 were owner-occupiers.

Table 3.2 Comparative tenure patterns

2001	England	Haringey	Bedford	Northamptonshire			
%				South	East	Kettering	Wellingborough
Owner occupied	68.9	45.8	72.4	79.2	76.2	76.9	72.3
Rented from local authority	13.2	19.7	1.4	9.5	4.3	10.8	16.2
Rented from housing association or registered social landlord	6.0	10.5	14.4	1.7	10.0	2.8	3.3
Private rented, or rent free	11.9	23.9	1.8	9.6	9.5	9.5	11.9

City, town or village?

In whichever size of settlement they were living, from the small village to the heart of metropolitan London, most of our respondents said that they were living in the place that was about right for them in terms of how urbanized it was. This may not be surprising: with settlement type as with housing itself, people may tend to move towards the comfortable and to become comfortable with the familiar. However, some people also expressed concerns or criticisms about the place where they lived and these were often related to levels of urbanization. Many of the respondents had experienced living in different kinds of places with which they could compare the place they were living now. For example, one Bedford resident described her strong affection for the countryside of her childhood, although she was very happy to now be living in the town with its convenience and activities:

> I used to go out in the fields with my granddad, this was when I was very young, I used to go out in the fields with my granddad and help him turn the hay, sit on the hay cart .... He had three horses, but he used to work a pair at a time. And I suppose with my whole life that is ... to the fore. I know it is the longest ago, but it is to the fore.
>
> I like it [here]. It is nice and open, it is right on the edge of town, but it is also close enough to nip into Bedford with no problem, apart from the buses [laughs]. ... Although I didn't know it when I came here, most of my neighbours are more or less in my own age group ... and they are very friendly. (Belinda)

In common with other studies of urban and rural life in the late 20th/

early 21st century, we found that respondents who lived in small settlements (villages and the smaller towns) were concerned about the loss
of public transport and amenities and opportunities for community
activities. By the same token, people who lived in Haringey generally had
fewer complaints about social or transport provision (with the excep-
tion, for some people, of accessibility). The Haringey residents were the
most dissatisfied with physical aspects of their environment (including
litter and 'dirt') even if they had no intention of moving. Respondents in
all sizes of settlement had things to say about social change and the
decline of community, including increasing crime. Nevertheless, most
respondents also were able to say positive things about their home if not
the location, to back up their conviction that it was better to stay where
they were than to move to another kind of place.

One of the differences between the locations was population density.
Our respondents lived with different degrees of closeness to their neighbours, ranging from those living in high density housing to the couple who
lived in a detached farm house just outside a village. One of them said:

> The country way of life bears no resemblance to the town .... And I
> couldn't live in a town ... not now. Because I can take the old dog for a
> walk on my own land and I don't have to worry whether it messes on the
> ground and whether I have to pick it up or not. (Norman)

For this man it was important to have space in both the literal sense
and in the sense of feeling free and unhindered by the concerns of
others. Yet it was clear that for other people living close to the countryside in villages or the smaller towns, the attraction of the 'green
environment' was complemented by the intimacy of 'village life', where
people expected to know something of each others' lives and to be
involved in active neighbouring. Cities are famously places where one
can be very socially active or very isolated in the anonymity of the
crowd; but clearly living cheek by jowl does not allow the physical
spaciousness needed by Norman. Many of our Haringey residents, like
respondents in the non-metropolitan locations, had good relationships
with particular neighbours and friends. However, they were much less
likely than the village dwellers to know much about most of their
immediate neighbours (for example, their names or something of their
history) and more likely on most days to see a lot of people that they
did not know at all.

Bedford, non-metropolitan yet large in comparison to the smaller towns and villages, was described by most of our respondents who lived there as a good place to live, despite its drawbacks. People here talked about local facilities and often of being able to walk to places in the town centre. The different areas of the town had been developed over a long time span and some of our respondents had specific attachments to their part of town:

> The neighbourhood fortunately is in a pleasant environment, it hasn't any . . . it has very limited numbers of people I should imagine are in the poverty trap. What I am saying to you, if you like to use the terms I don't like to use, they are lower middle class, or upper working class [laughs] they have got sufficient provisions to live a reasonable lifestyle, keep their properties in reasonably good attendance, the place looks reasonably clean. We do have the occasional vandalism, by students who might chop a tree down or do some damage. Apart from that it is kept in good order. Plus the local authorities also have a policy for keeping the verges cut and roads swept, and the trees trimmed if necessary. So all in all where I live I happen to have an excellent bus service every 10–15 minutes so that I can get to the town centre swiftly if I need to. I have a petrol station close to town, I have cinemas, dancing, and pubs galore. (Brian)

Belonging and change

> Well I suppose you can say I am a Burtoner folk now [laughs] I think I have been here long enough now, yes. (Nancy)

Nancy, whose experience is described in more detail in Chapter 7, regarded herself as one of the old guard of inhabitants who remember the town of Burton Latimer as it used to be: small, self-contained and communally minded. She was fairly unusual among the respondents in believing that the place where she lived belonged to her as much as she did to it. Most of our respondents had actually relocated several times and were now attached to the place where they lived, at least to the extent of not really wanting to live anywhere else. This sense of attachment related to networks of local support (kin, friends, neighbours) that could have an effect on how people lived their daily lives; and to their familiarity with the material environment. But respondents were generally more reticent about claiming 'belonging'. For many people, this concept appeared to imply a 'born and bred' insiderness that they could not claim even after many years of residence.

Change in communities and localities over time was a persistent theme, especially for people who had stayed put, regardless of the place or size of settlement. These changes included physical and social shifts ranging from the development of formerly green sites for 'executive' housing to the current ethnic mix of neighbourhoods:

> Bedford was a much better place before the war, and since after the war, but then immigration has been terrific with Italian brick workers, a big Italian community, Poles, oh umpteen nationals here now. But of course the Indians or Pakistanis they are everywhere, yes they are everywhere, they are the ones that have taken over all the shops of course. But Bedford used to be ... not an exaggeration to say that before the war, there was one coloured person in Bedford and he was very well known and he used to be a bus driver, and then I think he had his own taxi service, and he was very popular. There were others I think, there were Italians, but people came for the cheaper education, retired army people, but it was half the size it is now I should think. Quite a ... not tight community, you don't get to know people easily I don't think. Some people would call it snobbery I suppose, but I think it is just that people keep themselves to themselves more. But now of course at least half the people or more than that you meet are not Bedford people anyway. My wife wasn't, it took her a long while to settle in really, I think. She didn't know anybody when she came. I don't know if she had the same opinion about Bedford people as I did [laughs].

This contrasts with the experience of Belinda (quoted on page 63) who found her new neighbours in Bedford to be immediately friendly. Nevertheless themes of 'localness' and change in the ethnic and cultural composition of localities were found in both focus group discussions and in some of the respondents' personal accounts of area change. For example, members of one of the Haringey focus groups with mainly white participants commented that the high number of different languages and people of visibly different cultures sometimes made them feel alienated as they moved around the area, while a focus group of black-Caribbean residents discussed how they reacted to recent migrants from eastern Europe. In both cases the majority of people in these groups felt most concerned about the behaviour of young adults and children and about incidents of crime and disorder.

Crime and fear

In each of the locations, issues of crime and safety arose time and time again as people described how they used their neighbourhoods and what constrained their movements around them. Respondents in all areas gave examples of people they knew who had experienced crime or of their own experiences. These were often related to the neighbourhood change that we have already discussed and which in many, though not all cases, was experienced as unsettling. This respondent compared the Hornsey borough of old with the same district, now part of the borough of Haringey:

> I mean the streets were swept and the dustman came regular and it was a nice, clean tidy place ... I used to walk up the road three times a week to the bank for the shop, Mondays, Wednesdays, and Fridays and come with the change for the tills in a blue bag on my shoulder, never thought that I would be mugged and taken that off you. Go up the road with £2000 in your pocket and never thought you were going to be mugged in any way at all. No, it was a nice time then, against today's problems. I have just had my car busted in. (Harry)

And in the following extract, a respondent describes an incident that had a strong effect on her ability to get out and about after dark in her own neighbourhood. We relate the whole incident because it shows fairly graphically how an older individual's confidence can be undermined by a seemingly trivial episode.

> I suppose it was in April just before I was ill and I had to come home by bus ... and [as] I walked up ... I was very conscious of somebody following me. And I wouldn't look around, but I got quite het up within and I crossed over ... and I felt the footsteps coming nearer and nearer. And I couldn't resist it, I turned around, I had to you know, and it was a fellow. So I went on walking and suddenly he brushed past me, just touched my arm and said 'you needn't be so scared, I am only going home' and it was a young man. He didn't do anything, he just brushed past. ... Whether he intended doing anything or not and decided not to ... I don't know. But you see until then I never thought about it, but ever since then it has just left me with that uneasy feeling .... And you see there was not a soul around, it was just before midnight, there wasn't a soul around, only a fence down the bottom, there was no house there when I crossed over, there was nobody who could have come anywhere

near to help me, if he had decided to mug me. I had a handbag of course
.... I didn't know the man. But it was a very uneasy feeling. And it has
left me, this is the trouble, it has left me, I suppose I was lucky and got
away with it, but another time it could happen. So [today] I thought 'I
must get these two letters in the post' and so I went in the car, which is
ridiculous because it is only around the corner, and the walk would have
done me good, but I thought 'no, I am not walking round there'. It is
such a shame because we never used to feel like that, did we? (Helen)

It is generally recognized by policymakers that the fear of crime
expressed by older people far exceeds the likelihood of an individual
older person becoming the victim of crime and that this fear has
dramatic effect on how and when older people are prepared to venture
out into the community. This is not to say that all older people are
immobilized by fear and for the most part people in our study did get
out during daylight hours in spite of incidents; for example, members
of one focus group in Haringey talked about walking through insalu-
brious streets to get the shops, in spite of recent 'muggings' including
that of a very elderly neighbour. Nevertheless, the findings of several of
the projects in the ESRC Growing Older programme support the view
that fear of crime does have a negative effect (Holland et al., 2005) (see
also Age Concern, 2003) and a range of initiatives have been suggested
to overcome this problem, frequently focusing on combating media
over-representation of the risks and educating older people about
personal safety and the realities of crime patterns.

However, the older people we spoke to recognized where they had
control in relation to risk and safety both inside and outside their
homes. They felt unable to have much influence on the behaviour of
other people and some of them felt that their control of their own
bodies was compromised by disabilities or illnesses. The consequences
for them of, for example, a fall caused by a street crime or indeed the
damage to confidence described earlier by Helen, were potentially very
high. In making the risk assessment, they were balancing a low probability of harm against a high probability of serious consequences
should something happen to them. What they could control was their
own behaviour and they did this by evaluating places and their own
ability to keep out of danger. In this light the defensive behaviour of
many of our respondents within the world outside their homes appears
to be much more rational that the image of the unreasonably fearful

older person. It also helps to explain in part why they can, on the one hand, express a fear of going out into their neighbourhoods at night and, on the other hand, express attachment to those same neighbourhoods. As their assessment is usually that other places are just as bad if not worse, the fear of crime almost stands in isolation from other factors that our respondents took into account when describing their relationships with their neighbourhoods. Yet given the contradictions between identification with place and community and the prevalence of worries about change and disorder, how can older people maintain a sense of community?

Neighbourhoods and the sense of community

What do we mean by communities? Taylor et al. (2000) suggested that most communities can be defined by the common beliefs, economic status and activities of their populations and by the common interests that tie members together; while Etzioni (1995) wrote of the 'social webs of people who know one another as persons and have a "moral" voice'. Living in the same location is not necessarily a defining characteristic of communities. Indeed religious and cultural diaspora may span continents. Characteristics that give belonging to certain communities may implicitly exclude people from others. Ratcliffe (1999) and Alibhai-Brown (2000) have cited race, class, culture and economic status as such characteristics. Individuals may in fact align themselves with different groups and to varying degrees depending on the context they find themselves in. For example, the same person might wish to identify himself in response to different situations as a Bedford man, a grandfather, a retired civil servant or a British Muslim. The roles and status of individuals are not static and because they have lived for a long time older people in particular are likely to have experienced changes in how they relate to the wider community. For many older people, this has implications about their inclusion or exclusion in the life of the community.

For some people, including many older people, the reality is that day-to-day interactions with other people, especially in person, are confined to the immediate neighbourhood (if not entirely to their own home in the case of people who are housebound) and for many of our respondents these communities based on neighbourhood were essential to their well-being and sense of identity. Neighbourhoods, as distinct from communities, are geographical areas with personal and social meaning related to the physicality of the environment. Taylor and Brower (1985) describe them as those environments most proximate to individuals' homes in which interest and control are shared among households. Of course, this shared area includes many different kinds of place including those that may be regarded as private, semi-private and semi-public, and we go into these aspects in more detail in Chapter 4. In some cases it is possible to identify a bounded locality which is administratively or geographically defined (for example, a particular housing estate). But despite being geographically based, the definition of where a neighbourhood begins and ends is often far from simple and as experienced by individuals, boundaries are negotiable. They may include fixed elements (rivers; railway lines; main roads) but they may also be vague or undefined. For the purposes of studying identity and well-being, we defined an individual's neighbourhood as extending from their own front door to the point at which they felt they were 'out of the neighbourhood' – this usually meant that they no longer felt that they specifically belonged, or were known, or were deeply familiar with the physical environment.

Moving around

Moving around their own neighbourhoods, our respondents negotiated and interpreted the location as they engaged with the various elements of which it was composed. The material environment itself might be (relatively) simple and composed of few elements. For example, one of the larger sheltered housing schemes was composed of levels of similar flats, presenting views of either an internal courtyard or a rather unprepossessing mixed housing estate, so that for many residents with mobility problems the sheltered housing scheme had become in effect their whole neighbourhood. Alternatively, the neighbourhood might be highly complex with some aspects presenting barriers to social engagement; for example, a network of multiple-use streets.

Ageing and disability can entail a heightening of the sensual impact of the micro-environment, as material elements such as ground textures, changes in level and physical barriers become more problematic. Once personal mobility begins to diminish, the ability to move around and in and out of the immediate neighbourhood requires planning and strategy. Some people, especially older women, have never driven or have not had independent access to a car and certainly a few of our respondents still fell into this category. People who do drive are more likely to give up driving as they become older. The ability to get out beyond the immediate neighbourhood then requires accessible public transportation, taxis or the help of others. The sense of control over movement and mobility is crucial to self-esteem (Holland et al., 2005) and although most of our respondents in theory had people they could ask for lifts, in practice they tended to avoid 'bothering' people unless absolutely necessary.

Social neighbourhood

The complexity of social environments also varies from place to place. For example the range of socioeconomic classes present or the combination of minority ethnic groups and the extent to which these groups are integrated or segregated, differed among the locations that we studied. At all stages of life, people constantly edit their understanding of the social environment and construct networks of relationships based on opportunities and constraints on their own participation. During the period of our study (the turn of the 21st century) the context for these networks was an increasingly complex society and the 20th century had seen smaller households, more geographically dispersed families, more people living alone for extended periods including later life and a move away from pre- and post-war collectivism in social activities towards more privatism and privatization. Some of the respondents reflected on these changes, usually in the context of regret about social cohesion, even though few specifically said that they wanted more interaction with their neighbours than they currently had:

> By and large when I look around not only our own neighbourhood, we tend to build big fences around each other and hide away behind them, and I think that is very sad. People have become very security conscious. They think that by building a big wall they are safer, they are not really. (Bernard)

Place in time

Interpreting the neighbourhood also carries a time dimension. Collective memories and stories about aspects of the neighbourhood contribute to the 'insiderness' of people familiar with neighbourhood histories. For example, among our respondents who were long-term residents some occasionally referred to places by historic or arcane names or gave directions by referring to landmarks that had long been removed. They could also recollect the notable events, personal or collective, that had happened in specific locations. Familiar places, especially those with which people have longstanding involvements, can support older people in a number of ways. These include under-writing an 'entitlement' to place because of a co-history of habitation; and giving people the security of knowing other people and being known by them, if only by sight. It also gives the confidence of knowing how to handle the material environment – good places to cross the road, the location of public lavatories, shortcuts, safe routes and places to avoid. Walking round her village in the company of Nullah, we were struck by her constant narrative as she related parti-cular places to particular events and people, so that for her a whole social history of the village was mapped out in its physical terrain.

Yet memories alone are not enough. People also need current knowledge about their neighbourhoods to be able to negotiate and interpret them. Familiarity can give confidence and one of the problems with other people's neighbourhoods is the uncertainty about interpreting their spaces. How people actually use that knowledge to act within their neighbourhoods is related to life stage, opportunities, expectations and the extent to which people feel accepted (and not under a critical gaze) or fearful or anxious when they are out and about. For some older people, security concerns can result in an involuntary disengagement from the neighbourhood although in the case of our respondents this was pri-marily temporal and after dark. Others find a solution in what has been described as the 'integrated segregation' of communities of older people (McGrail et al., 2001). We go on to discuss settings specifically for older people in Chapter 6. Such communities, in recreating a secure internal neighbourhood, may also reinforce the 'otherness' of older people rela-tive to the wider population (Phillips et al., 2001). The tension between comfort and discomfort in neighbourhoods has emerged as an important theme in understanding older people's constructions of home.

Getting involved

Attachment to place, at whatever level, requires some element of personal identification and we have remarked on the fact that many respondents remained attached, in theory at least, to places that were far distant or where they had not visited for many years. Yet to remain attached to the neighbourhood all of those who touched on this topic were agreed that a proper relationship with it requires some active involvement. Indeed, it was one of the common criticisms of modern society that people generally and younger people in particular seem to have lost sight of the importance of local involvement:

> They don't ... there is a community here, but it is a different type of community. It is 'we will do it if we can' but sometimes it is 'we will do it if there is nothing better to do' and that is putting it rather brutally. People are out all day, and by the time they come home in the evening perhaps it is 8–9.00 pm something like that. But we led pretty busy lives, so keeping your family, and you certainly didn't have the help you have today. ...
>
> There is still no end to what we could do down there, but it is the manpower and cash really to improve the environment down there. And it takes time, and so few people these days want to volunteer, you know. 'oh I haven't got time, I am busy' and I say 'well so am I but I still find time to contribute a bit to the community' which is what it is about isn't it? (Nullah)

Everyone in our study except those living in residential care homes had some level of involvement with their local community, ranging from shopping locally and a weekly appointment with a social club, to being a local councillor. The previous quotes show something of the importance that many of our respondents placed on interactivity with the world outside their own homes. For the more mobile, getting out of the house and into the wider community of the city, town or village was an essential part of continuing to feel alive and connected:

> Yes. I can't sit in the house, I have got to be up and doing something, I go for walks, I go into the town, I wonder around the town and I come here and play snooker with the guys, I go and talk with some of the inmates, members. I have got to know by going around the town most of the staff in most of the stores, just having a chat with them, and it is nice, a nice feeling. I get myself known around the neighbourhood. It is how you get yourself known, I think it is important for the neighbourhood to get together a bit more. (Bernard)

Getting involved was also a strong theme in discussions about relocations and getting settled in a new place; and in discussions about adjusting to widowhood. Some of the respondents, particularly those who had moved many times during their lives, appeared to have been particularly adept at making new friends wherever they found themselves. Those with strong bonds to established churches said that they had been able to make friends fairly quickly through the church: the larger established religions form aspatial communities of interest, in which it can be argued that the 'minority' identity as co-religionist is stronger than the ageing one. However, it must be stated here that the nature of our study precluded the involvement of reclusive people. All our respondents could draw, to a greater or lesser extent, on social capital.

Conclusion

We have tried to show in this chapter that location matters. The experience of our respondents includes environment at all levels from the global perspective of migrants and travellers to the nuanced micro environments of places within rooms. At the levels we have considered here, the material and social elements of identifiable places have become part of the fabric from which they have created their identities. For some people the town or part of the city is an essential part of the story – another home could be contemplated, but it would have to be in this place. For others, the home itself is the anchor and the attachments to location are more functional than emotional. For everyone the kind of place in terms of size, social mix, civic pride, natural environment, urbanization etc. must be accounted for in their description of where they currently are as a person.

Many countries face change brought about by globalization, environmental change, changing social structures, increasing longevity and declining birth rates and developments in forms of communication and technologies. Yet in terms of interaction at the practical and everyday level, it is the neighbourhood that continues to be the more significant point of attachment to society for most older people. The neighbourhood provides a context for and a bridge between the intimacy of the dwelling place and the wider public domains of township/county/state/country – with any or all of which people might identify at some level, but not really know in the intimate way that they know their neighbourhood. No longer being able to go out independently is therefore a critical stage in identity construction because, without the wider contexts that lie beyond the dwelling, the home itself becomes diminished as a source of identity construction. Continued capacity to engage with 'the other' is represented by neighbourhood in a way that the immediate domicile cannot demonstrate or provide.

Neighbourhood deterioration, by affecting the ways that older people can interact in those places that are close to home, therefore has a particularly profound effect on the lives of older people. The rate of neighbourhood change, as well as its nature, is crucial to whether people can feel in control; rapid change can disrupt the congruence between personal identity and the place identity that is an important part of attachment to place.

Given that individuals react differently to their environments, and environments have different effects on people, can we begin to identify the kinds of neighbourhoods that are most likely to help older people to remain socially engaged? How inclusive can the locality of neighbourhood be for people in later life? Some older people can still rely on support from within neighbourhoods (see studies by Phillipson et al. of Bethnal Green, Wolverhampton and Woodford (2001)). Many of our respondents are themselves supportive and active neighbours. Yet most of them have very few neighbours that they would actually feel comfortable about calling on for help except in an emergency. The study has shown us that alongside trans-spatial engagements with family and wider communities through technology (telephone/television/internet), *actual* engagement in the material and social neighbourhood is still essential to well-being and self-identity. To date neighbourhood has been relatively underemphasized in considering optimal environments for older people, yet it is clear that as people age and may become more focused on home, the salience of neighbourhood is likely to increase. In Britain, most people as they age remain in 'regular' neighbourhoods rather than move into collective retirement communities. It remains one of the great challenges of our ageing society to make those neighbourhoods good places in which to grow old and in which older people can continue to contribute.

Notes

1 Bedford Development Association, 2003.

2 These are Corby BC; Daventry DC; Kettering BC; Northampton BC; Wellingborough BC; and the Councils of East Northamptonshire and South Northamptonshire.

3 Mid-census data from local authorities.

4

Thresholds

Surroundings

In Chapter 4, we move from the street and the wider community to the gardens, the yards, the grassed surroundings and pathways, the balconies and porches and windows of 'ordinary' and 'special' housing. Places that may be tended or cultivated or purposeful space that can be used for watching, sitting, eating, reading, hanging washing, tending much loved flowers or institutional floral borders, walking, playing, parking vehicles, leaving refuse: all activities within spatial areas that are attached to accommodation, but often under-researched.

We have reached the point of crossing the threshold into the more personal territory that marks the divide between the wider neighbourhood and the 'home space'. The exteriors and surrounds of all forms of housing can give an impression of their occupants: for many older people this will include mainstream housing where they have lived for more than 20 years (Lindberg et al., 1992). In his book on the psychology of home Gunter (2000) comments: 'The home serves as a reflection on how we want to see ourselves and be seen by others'. Our home is thus 'an extension of our personalities' (Haywood, 1977, p.12). The validity of this statement varied for those who took part in our study. Many have lived in their present home for a long time and have a sense of how they wish to be seen, the activities they wish to participate in and what they wish to observe. Others have moved more recently and while some have re-engaged with their current accommodation and location to see it as a basis for forward planning, others may be less able to see the 'extension of their own personalities' within their new environment. Here we focus on how the surroundings of accommodation may influence identity.

Defining surroundings involves a number of aspects. As seen in Chapter 1, Rowles, through detailed biographical research, considered the experience of older people in terms of both space and place, defining domains in which both 'personal' and 'specific' experiences can be located. In his terms, we are now concerned with the 'surveillance zone'; watchful space from the house (Rowles, 1981). However, through examination of the 'Environment and Identity' data, the 'surveillance zone' is extended to encompass that space external to accommodation and forming a 'buffer zone' with the wider society. Here two distinct aspects of this liminal space are identified: *first*, enclosed external space – garden, yard, balcony – bounded by fence/shrubs/path/railings to define territory that is the domain of those who live or work within the accommodation that may be called 'home'. This is space that may be entered either from the private space of the housing/accommodation or from the public space of the drive or street. It is seen as 'defensible space' for the occupant of mainstream housing and even more so by home owners, as people are able to control to different degrees who they invite in (Newman, 1973; Gunter, 2000). And *second*, space that could be called 'tended and watchful space' relates to internal space that may allow a degree of cultivation through the use of flowers, plants, window boxes on sills and ledges that enable people to engage with a version of the natural environment that can be potted and transported. It also relates to the external environment as seen or heard from windows/doors/patios (part of the accommodation) – extending the gaze beyond 'owned' space and on to other public and private thoroughfares and territories.

Expectations of settings

We have already noted the cross-setting focus of this research and so before examining how interaction with the immediate environment may impact on individual identity it is helpful to reconsider the location and personal histories of the 'Environment and Identity' respondents. Research on the 'ideal' home from the late 1990s (Popular Housing Forum, 1998) shows that people in younger and middle-age groups prefer to live in quiet locations that are close to amenities in a 'nice area', and that space around the house and security are important features. While these preferences also exist among our respondents, they may to some extent reflect generational experiences and differing societal expectations. For example, older people who have spent their lives as flat dwellers in the city or town may never have experienced a personal garden; while for others the experience of gardening has been acquired over time. For Harry, the experience of being involved with a garden came with the development of council housing that provided many working-class families with a garden for the first time. In his interview he talks of housing that he lived in with his family during the inter-war period:

> [U]ntil they found us another council house at Ilford, Essex. It was a pre-war council house this one, but of course very, very nice, bathroom and toilet and front and back gardens. And that sort of thing. (Harry)

One can hear the pleasure at having amenities in this comment, and 'front and back gardens' can infer a level of status that may not have been experienced before. In contrast, Neenah had spent her childhood living in the grounds of a large estate in a tied house where her father had been head gardener. She liked sitting out in the large garden of her present home but expressed no interest in gardening herself and was happy to leave it to her husband.

The social production of such amenities relates to historical and cultural understandings of family accommodation and institutional settings (Townsend, 1962; Willcocks et al., 1987; Peace, 1993). The space surrounding, or siting, different forms of accommodation is seen as both a private and a public utility. These historical comments by planners reflect a diversity of understandings that may have influenced the design of environments in which our respondents have lived:

> The post-war improvements in the standard of living mean that few families now rely on the garden to keep them properly fed. It is now used for outdoor living, for children's play and the baby's sleep; and it is cultivated either for the pleasure of gardening or only because it has to be kept tidy . . . . In all gardens arrangements are required which will ensure a reasonable degree of privacy for sitting out and having meals outside. Present day gardens are often sadly lacking in this amenity. (MHLG, 1961, p.39)

In contrast, the residential care home for older people has not been seen as a place for individual pursuits but as a place of work and where older people are thought to need something interesting to look at:

> Sites should be reasonably level. Access to roads and public transport and
> to ordinary amenities of town or village life – shops, post offices,
> churches and places of entertainment – should be easy and distances
> short. An interesting aspect is important: backland sites and lifeless
> prospects should be avoided. Safe access to the building for cars,
> ambulances and vans and space for parking, turning and delivery will be
> required. It is especially important that account should also be taken of
> the need for staff to get to their homes or places of entertainment easily.
> (DHSS, 1973, pp.2–3)

Comments from these policy documents reflect a particular period
and display an ongoing difference between accommodation that is seen
as domestic and that seen as non-domestic, which constitutes the
current range of accommodation for respondents in the present study.
In particular the 1973 quotation from the DHSS in outlining the
varying needs of the surroundings of these forms of accommodation as
places of work identifies the power base of institutional settings. The
tension between the needs of the individual and the collective can also
be seen in the development of sheltered housing. While many people
may identify giving up the responsibility of a garden as one reason for
moving (Heywood et al., 2002, p.82), a small number of tenants will
make a request for a ground-floor apartment that has access to a small
garden area.

We wanted to consider what meanings our older respondents give to
these different forms of space and how these meanings might influence
the ways that people identity with a place. Our respondents' understanding of these spaces forms a social construction revealed in stories
of everyday routines, memories and actions (Lefebvre, 1991; Hayden,
1995). To begin we reflect on the importance of the natural environment to the ways in which the respondents said they felt about
themselves.

Importance of nature

The juxtaposition between natural and material environments becomes
central to this discussion. While 'home' is seen as a refuge and a place
of protection, research also shows the preference for an open view from
accommodation that may allow people to see who is coming to visit

them and activities in their surroundings (Nasar, 1983; Nasar et al., 1989). Symbolic meaning is also noted in the preference for naturalness through greenery, trees and vegetation in both urban and rural locations, where it is associated with feelings of well-being (Kaplan, 1985; Kaplan and Kaplan, 1989; Ulrich et al., 1991). Such a view is reflected in the following comment:

> But the thing was it was a low block, six floors downside, and from the view of Tottenham ... we had this balcony at the back and the front, looking across Tottenham there were these unusual trees, the closed nunnery, which is now a Muslim educational centre, there was the parish church a beautiful outlook. And from the rear balcony we had this lovely garden and a willow tree. And in the 10 years the willow had been stripped by the children in the area, you know [whispering]. We had prostitutes at the front of the building. And the front of the building just changed because of stripping down trees and putting up flats. And actually to see the willow tree stripped made me cry, it sounds awful, but it did it made me feel really sad, and I found myself calling over the balcony 'don't destroy the tree' which of course made them do it all the more. But whatever they did to the garden, overnight it had been destroyed. And the little park where we used to take the dogs for a walk they had destroyed the play area there, the swings, the clubhouse was all burnt overnight. But I have always, wherever I have been, I have always managed to find ... because I love birds, I always found something pleasant to look at you know, to compensate the bits that I don't like. I suppose we all do. (Hermione)

Here, one of the respondents living in Haringey captures, in her reflections on past housing, tensions between individual and collective identity. As a woman of 72 years she has watched city development and what she considers cultural decline change the landscape, prompting her to recognize her own values and reconfirm the importance of the natural environment to her own well-being. Her comments reveal the ways in which the contrast between the material and the natural environments can be central and ongoing to the lives of anyone wherever they may live: 'I have always found something pleasant to look at you know, to compensate the bits that I don't like.'

These comments demonstrate how the natural environment can have profound meanings for individuals in any location. Our three locations were metropolitan, urban/suburban and semi-rural areas in southeast England and consequently the proximity and immediacy of the natural environment whether it be garden space, open vistas or trees along a street varied. The interview data were examined through content analysis of key themes relating to gardens, yards, plants, trees, flowers, birds, walls, fences, paths and while it is true that most respondents living in Northamptonshire commented on the natural environment and fewer did in Haringey, there is not an extreme difference (see Table 4.1). Indeed previous research has shown that the presence of the natural environment can increase people's enjoyment of the urban environment with vegetation 'an antidote to many of the physical ills of the city' (Gunter, 2000, p.28) (Kaplan and Kaplan, 1989; Ulrich et al., 1991). A review of research on natural landscapes in urban areas, sponsored by English Nature (Rohde and Kendle, 1994) documents the value of nature for emotional sustenance, feelings of calm, serenity and restoration as well as exhilaration.

However, when analyzing data from the 54 respondents in the in-depth study, it is apparent that certain characteristics may have influenced their comments. As we have seen many people had lived at their present address for a long time, at least 20 years, and both housing/accommodation type and ownership influenced this discussion enabling some respondents to see their environs as a part of themselves. Housing tenure and consequent control over territory and choice of use varied – from the owner-occupier of domestic housing with access to a garden at both the front and back of the building; to the tenant of a flat with a balcony accessed through French windows; to the resident of a sheltered housing apartment able to walk to a seat within a protected quadrangle at the centre of the building.

Close examination of the narratives also shows how aspects of the immediate environs can be seen in different ways. A couple living in a farmhouse in Northamptonshire had found that this setting supported the wife, who had long-term mental health problems, by not being intrusive. Here there is a sense of protection. They spoke together of their joy in country living that they would not wish to lose:

A: I would feel very lost if I couldn't see green fields out of one of my windows you see, from out there. I like to be in the countryside quickly.

B: Well, we had someone come the other day and they looked

Table 4.1 Comments relating to the natural environment

Location	Yes	No
Haringey	11	7
Bedford	13	5
Northamptonshire	17	1

Total Numbers of Respondents N = 54

out the back and said 'oh you are in the country really now'.

A: Squirrels in the garden, yes. Foxes are here.

[*Interviewer*: Would you ever contemplate moving to a small house, or a bungalow, or a place with a small garden?]

A: No, I don't think so, no.

B: I would find it very hard if I couldn't open that door and go into the garden. I would hate to live in a flat when all I have got to do is sit in a park. Very hard.
             I was thinking we ought to move, but I don't think it is on, I like it too much and . . . it is the only place she has ever lived since we have been married, with this illness, that she has been happy. (Ned & Wife)

The comments made here are about rural living and the 'buffer zone' is something all-embracing that allows this couple to adopt a particular lifestyle.

In discussing the meaning of home respondents from all three locations talked about being out of doors and the importance of space and vista. There is a sense that greenery may be health enhancing by making people feel good about themselves (Gunter, 2000). Hilary, a 61-year-old woman from Barbados who came to the UK as a nurse in 1970, spent much of her younger life living in nurses' hostels before buying a house in Tottenham with her former husband. She now shares the house with her grown-up sons. Her life has not been uneventful and in conversations she talks about her life in the West Indies, which has given her a different experience of space. Her comments disclose both a need to find peace and soak up the calm of the external space and a desire to establish her own order within a situation (both internal and external) over which she sometimes does not feel in total control. Her ownership of this space is important to her well-being. She comments:

> When my sons are here with their friends I just close the door, I have my garden, I like my garden looking out ...
>
> I hope to get cracking ... I walk past there every day, if there is a plant dying I sort of adopt that plant and take it. And I went home and tried to get it better, some people like animals and I like plants. And I like the garden. And you will be surprised to know, for the first time I really splashed out, I went to Homebase and I ordered a ... where you sit down ... and the picnic bench was only £27, so I thought 'oh, I will have a picnic bench and we can have a cup of tea outside' and it was still there in the box because two days after they were delivered, I brought the wood preserve and everything, two days after, I was at home and got a call from my mother saying that she had a cataract, and so I forgot about that completely and went ... I have got somewhere to park my car. I haven't got a car ... never had one [laughs]. But you can sit here and count your blessings. You can sit here and there is nobody looking over us, I am not over looking any other houses, you see. You can sit here and know that there is nobody looking at us, you know that. See those trees. (Hilary).

Indeed for some of our urban respondents, access to external space gained from a doorway to a yard could give a feeling of extended space:

> Well, being on the ground floor you have got ... well they have got the wire fencing back but the kids have broken it down again. And so I have got the doorway there ... so that little bit there, I had to make a garden like that to stop the kids, cats, and dogs. So I had that much breathing space, because if I didn't I would choke. (Hester)

Gardening

The garden has long been seen as the place for restoring the self (Kaplan and Kaplan, 1987). Analysis of the focus group data from the first stage of the study shows that across all the locations, the use of gardens, enjoyment of gardening, and the problems of not being able to maintain a garden, were common to all discussions. This was a discussion of the cultivated environment rather than rural living and some respondents commented on the importance of the physical nature of the garden when choosing their present accommodation:

But the thing that attracted us was the garden really, and the bungalow generally. We did quite a bit to it, it was somewhat neglected before we came and we wanted to get it more or less how we wanted it. (Barry)

It is obvious that this is a crucial factor in both the maintenance of 'staying put' and later decisions concerning moving that will be discussed in Chapter 6. Here, we focus first on the ways in which the garden can become a part of the 'natural me':

A garden can provide for other important needs. One view is that it serves to bring us into closer contact with nature. The attraction of plants and greenery has been described as being 'almost primordial' – a genetic imprint dating from prehistory when vegetation was essential to human survival (Kron, 1983). Keen gardeners also obtain gratification from an encounter with nature that produces tangible outcomes. (Kaplan, 1973)

A house with a garden has what almost amounts to an extended 'personality', an additional dimension which affords occupants the potential for extra fulfilment from their home. (Gunter, 2000, pp.24–25, 27–28)

Cultivating a garden was important to some people and keen gardeners were found in all locations. The garden was discussed in a number of ways: for some gardening was a lifelong interest and for others it had become an interest on retiring from paid work. The garden could also be a 'talking point' enabling them to display their expertise.

[S]he did manage the garden very well considering she was what I call a 'flower person' and I am a 'vegetable person'. (Barbara)

Where respondents had lived in a house for a very long time, the garden generated feelings beyond skill or sentiment and reflected a family history full of personal meaning. This statement by Nerys situates people in place and demonstrates the attachment that such connections involve:

There is quite a lot in the garden … it has quite a lot of personal memories … the little rose bush at the bottom, it's a florabunda, my eldest daughter bought it at Woolworth's and her daddy put it in a long time ago and it blossoms and it's always known as Dawn's tree, Dawn's rose because she actually put it in. (Nerys)

In contrast, others described the garden as a functional setting for social activities where people could interact and which had to be made presentable; but it was not necessarily central to their lives beyond this sense of order:

> I just enjoy the house, enjoy the garden. I quite often sit out there in the nice weather, it is very nice you know ... I like to see a nice garden, but I don't do a lot, bits and pieces you know, but I am not a good gardener, no. (Harry)

However, a maintained and ordered environment was important for giving people a sense of pride and commitment to their home, which was also important in reflecting their own identity. It is interesting to note that few of the respondents talked about maintaining the accommodation itself through tasks such as painting.

Comment on 'front and back gardens' also identifies the changing nature of spatial type along a spectrum of public and private space. The nature of this space as more or less public or private will be reflected in different types of behaviour, learned rather than instinctive, which can affect levels of and type of individual, family and group activity and meaning. For example, a front garden may be experienced as semi-public as people converse with those walking along a street from behind the protection of their own walled garden or chat to neighbours over a wall as this woman commented:

> I talk over the garden, next door I am always chatting to her, she is Italian. If I see her in the garden or meet her in the street we have a chat, we get on alright. And this one here, she has got three children but they are all grown up and gone now, so she only has one son with her at the moment and a grandson, something like that. (Helen)

Contrariwise, taking a meal or sitting and relaxing is more usual in the privacy of the rear of the accommodation. Here a man interviewed in a residential care home where he was currently living for a period of rehabilitation, talks of how his own front garden deliberately draws attention to itself:

> Oh, you ought to see my front garden, I have got all little ornaments there that I put down. And all the children come down from the high school, and they take photos and notes, and everything. And the junior school, they come down and other people come down with big cameras and take photos of it.

And I have got a plate out there 'home sweet home' on a plate. I got Laurel and Hardy which I made out of plastics. I have got dogs, and little rabbits, and things I have done, you know. (Horace)

These comments demonstrate a form of attachment that differs fundamentally from that seen in shared garden or yard space surrounding flats, maisonettes or 'special' housing. Here, ownership is important for there is something about the ability to control what occurs within this space that makes it very different from the street or the interior of the home and how it is perceived (Shlay, 1985). The material and natural environment from which this space is created is important. Location affects meaning, which will continue to be constructed and reconstructed in different ways.

The 12 respondents who lived in residential care homes or sheltered housing were the least likely to comment on the immediate external environment. It can be argued that the needs for shelter, security and companionship are more pressing, although it is also true that these respondents had less opportunity to maintain or develop any gardening activities. While those residents in residential care homes were not involved in any external gardening, residents in sheltered housing were in a different position. While all the sheltered housing tenants could use a communal garden, those living in ground-floor apartments were sometimes able to access a small garden area via a French window or other door. Some members of our focus groups had taken advantage of this opportunity to make their own mark on the tiny area outside their windows. In one of the Haringey settings, a focus group resident took us to see her patio garden and told us of the pleasure that she took in tending and watering plants – a slow, planned task but one that gave her great enjoyment.

Gardens: a form of environmental press?

The question posed as to whether older people are 'prisoners of space' (Rowles, 1978) leads to a consideration of people's interactions with and mastery over their immediate environment. Through it they can become visible or invisible, concealed or revealed. When examining interactions with immediate surroundings, we find that Goffman's work on the presentation of self continues to have application (1959). In considering 'region behaviour', he utilized the theatrical discourse to consider settings of performance distinguishing between 'front' and 'back' regions where people's actions may be revealed or concealed. He makes this comment in relation to 'front regions': 'The performance of an individual in the front region may be seen as an effort to give the appearance that his activity in the region maintains and embodies certain standards' (1959, p.110). Such standards relate to rules and codes by which people behave, to the respect that is shown for a 'region' and the order that is maintained. Failure to maintain such standards or appearances may lead others to question the person's independence or for them to feel increasingly insecure. In contrast 'back regions' allow the person to 'relax; he can drop his front, forgo speaking his lines, and step out of character' (Goffman, 1959, p.115). These are places for what Goffman calls 'impression management' and this distinction has direct application for a discussion of the spaces that provide a 'buffer zone' and can be seen as semi-public or semi-private (Gregson and Rose, 2000) where permission for 'entering' and 'leaving' can be controlled.

Gardens at the front and the back of housing are of particular interest. People adopt different forms of behaviour within these difference locations and the very nature of gardens can act as an indicator of maintaining standards. Grass that gradually becomes overgrown and flower beds no longer the pride and joy of the gardener, may begin to reveal that the occupant of the housing is no longer coping with this task. It may be that a wife or husband has lost their partner who was always the gardener. It may be that preserving energy to maintain the home means that the outdoors must be neglected, not prioritized, relative to the inside as it does not necessarily impinge on daily life except through a concern for standards. Many older people call on family members to help with some aspects of basic gardening. Others, who have always enjoyed gardening as a pastime, will find other ways of continuing to garden through tending potted plants or reducing their work to a raised bed or rockery. Nancy, whose poor health has caused her to do less gardening, has been fortunate to find a neighbour who helps her:

> I love my garden it's just big enough for me, until I got osteoporosis and then I fractured my femur it was ... I could do it myself ... but I can't get down to do it now and me neighbour helps, he has to come and do it

now, it's very kind of him, so that gets done. I ... I've started putting things in pots and I can have a pot (around) meself. (Nancy)

Finding people to help is one way forward, while paying for help is another option if this can be afforded and help can be found:

A huge problem you know and we can't get anybody to come and help. Spoke to a lady last year who was doing gardens, big gardens, if she could take us on, she said she couldn't because she and her father were doing 30 gardens a week, cutting grass, haven't got time for it. So I am on my own right here. Just have to do a bit ... a lot of them have turned into bushes and things like that. Grass has to be cut. My son when he was 16 built the fishpond at the bottom of the garden. Now he's gone, I wouldn't have a fishpond, with fish and all that. So that's got to be cleaned out at least and looked after. So it keeps me busy, if I'm not in my garden, I am doing a bit of painting. (Neil)

Respondents living in Northamptonshire on the whole tended to have more garden space than those in either Bedford or Haringey, but access to help with gardens was a general concern and focus groups in Bedford in particular commented on the difficulty of finding anyone to take on this kind of work on a regular basis. Respondents in this position realized that their garden was becoming an issue that would have to be dealt with because it might identify them in some way as people who could not cope. This garden space, in becoming problematic, now presents a form of environmental press, as comments from several respondents show:

The garden didn't seem all that big when we first came, but it has got bigger as we got along .... The garden seems big now, and I would like to get some help with that because three years ago I wasn't very well and had an operation and some radiotherapy and ... in fact I am still waiting for more, I don't know yet, and I just don't seem to have the energy to cope with it. Also my son and grandson are very good, when they can they help out or sometimes he stays overnight and does a few jobs for me. (Barry)

Of course, finding someone to help means accepting someone else's standards:

And the garden is too big. But ... [*Interviewer:* Do you have any help?] No, No, What I said 'what would I do if I won the lottery?' what I would do, I would employ a gardener [laughs] and somebody said ... 'he would never do it right for you'. (Norman)

These comments may present classic examples for the application of Lawton's environmental docility hypothesis. However, the maintenance of the garden presents an interesting issue for there are varying levels of decline in relation to a garden depending on how far the person has adopted the role of the gardener as a part of their identity. If the person has always done the gardening themselves then the decline of the garden may highlight the individual's own physical decline and have direct impact on how they see themselves. However, where gardening has been a less essential task its decline may be 'kept at bay' or temporarily forgotten because it is external space where to some extent 'nature tends to itself'. Of course, here the difference in function between the back and front garden can come into play as the shabby nature of a neglected garden reveals itself. The level of family and other support may prove essential to developing a system of maintenance that enables the older person to maintain a level of self-respect in the presentation of their home and this can also depend on financial resources and, as we have indicated, the realistic availability of private assistance.

Vistas and cultivation indoors

The environment across the threshold that may only be seen from a window – 'watchful space' – can also allow people to observe flora, fauna and human activity throughout the seasons and across the days (Lewis, 1973). This may offer stimulation and give pleasure, enabling the individual to reach beyond their immediate concerns and physical limitations. This was true of Barbara, a woman now living in sheltered housing in Bedford, who describes how she can both concentrate on the changing life cycle of one particular tree and watch the birds, while also observing the routines of other people through her window:

> I think I am the only flat on the whole complex that has an uninterrupted view across the park. But I mean, the flat ... [previous location], it was just part of a huge complex of flats and we had no view at all, not really, well practically none, it was just a little bit of a view mainly looking into other flats. But then you learn to adapt and to appreciate little things.

Like we had a crab-apple tree outside one window, and you get to notice the detail. But then again this is the attitude, do you accept what you have got and learn to see what you can enjoy in it? Or do you fuss about what you haven't got [laughs]?

I tend to have my meals on a tray by the window so that I can watch the birds, that is when I notice the gentleman below that takes his wife over in the wheelchair to the [residential care home], I see them to-ing and fro-ing, I see a few people to-ing and fro-ing. And then, of course, occasionally, I see some of them getting around the garden, but you see people aren't all that mobile. (Barbara)

This level of engagement with the wider environment was also true for Bart, a 61-year-old man who had physical limitations following a stroke. He lived in a high-rise flat in Bedford and was especially interested in watching birds, having developed an interest in owls:

But apart from that I don't really go out at all. ... you know I don't like being on my own too much and if we have good weather I want to go to the marina. I go to my sister-in-law's ... for about three days because I am quite close to them. I call her sister, she was married to my brother. I am quite well with them, I go down for three days, we go to RSPB [Royal Society for the Protection of Birds], I see the owls. I had never seen an owl before, although we heard a tawny owl somewhere around here, and we have got a sparrowhawk owl somewhere around here as well. But I have got a bird box on my balcony, I have blue tits in. But that is about all I do. (Bart)

The natural environment and its cultivation continued to be important to many respondents for whom this had now become the tending of pot plants indoors. For some this was an indoor hobby and an extension of gardening outside, while for others certain plants held connections and meanings with life history. Harjit, Indian born, had lived in the UK for many years. He associated particular plants with herbal and religious customs. Now living in sheltered housing, he was no longer able to water the plants and relied on friends to cultivate them although he still saw these as a part of his indoor environment:

Oh yes, that is a temple plant there, which is from India, it is supposed to be good luck and goodness. The other one is a yucca, this one is an aromatic plant, and this one is supposed to be a money plant. My friends got it, they come in and tidy up every now and again they come and do it, every Monday, one of my friends comes and waters the plants and things like that. (Harjit)

For many people the presence of nature, wherever they live, is essential; for others it is a less obvious part of self – a background to be missed if it is not present (Kaplan and Kaplan, 1989; Nasar, 1989; Kuo et al., 1998). Attachment to place can be communicated through interaction within this 'buffer zone' of the home range; exemplified by the home owner who can recall the individual flowers planted as a long-time gardener; or the high-rise dweller for whom the inside/outside boundary has become the view from the window. The seasonality of the natural environment is symbolic of all that is growing, that will die, and that will be replenished and many older people draw comfort from it.

Boundaries and territoriality

People are often able to regulate the social distance between themselves and other people (Hediger, 1950; Hall, 1966) through control over the territory sometimes described as 'defensible space'. Personal and group identity can be derived from the ability to establish and maintain an area that is seen to symbolize belonging and this may have positive or negative affects in terms of well-being. Norman, a 69-year-old man living on a farm in rural Northamptonshire talks through the gains and losses implied in the prospect of selling off some of his land to enable him to 'stay put' – conveying feelings of ownership, independence and freedom:

Yes, but I don't want somebody living in my back doorstep particularly, unless I know them ... there could be somebody coming to convert one of those barns, somebody we have known ever since we have been here, and they would be an ideal neighbour.

We have always had neighbours until we came here, but it is nice not to have to worry about neighbours, what they are doing, whether they are having a party or whatever they are doing. That is it, that is life. And this is when you come to the crunch of it isn't it.

I would be satisfied if we took where the barn is, drew a line across there and say 'right up to that fence there that is your place, you can have that' that would suit me, because there is nothing that way and there is nothing that way. And it would be sufficient enough, perhaps I am just being unsociable, but there isn't much. I don't think we have much choice. (Norman)

Feelings about surroundings

In Chapter 1, we saw that when discussing 'feelings' Rowles (1978) considered issues of permanence and association that demonstrate the emotional quality that some people may associate with specific spaces. While this interpretation of feelings may be used in relation to all aspects of the environment, our analysis of the environment between accommodation and street begins to show the different ways in which personal identity can be witnessed through levels of interaction that demonstrate an engagement with a wider natural and material environment and that may or may not involve physical activity.

In summary, our analysis of the data from the 'Environment and Identity' study relating to surroundings, focuses on three areas that show how environment may influence the construction of identity in later life. These are the importance of the natural environment physically, aurally and visually, and its impact on attachment to place; second, the way in which the presence of this surrounding space may lead to an increased recognition of engagement and disengagement that impacts on personal identity as people grow older; and, finally, the relationship between territoriality and autonomy that encourages confidence in the self.

5

Homing In

One aspect of the ways in which people engage with others involves the consideration of whether or not to reveal aspects of the self. To do this people construct and reconstruct their biography for themselves in order to present a face to the world. We have seen how subtly and selectively these processes can be played out beyond the boundaries of the home, and in the gardens, balconies and windows of observed/observable space. In this chapter, we consider how older people draw on the interior of their homes to explain – again to self, and to others – who and what they are and what they have done and continue to do in the world. The mainstream domestic environment can also be used to conceal aspects of self and for older people this may well include covering up increasing levels of frailty.

In the 'Environment and Identity' cross-setting study, we find people living alone and in couples, in mainstream housing, and in settings that have been specially designed for older people (see Figure 5.1).

The gradient from mainstream housing through to the most specialized environments (residential homes in terms of the respondents in focus here, although nursing homes are probably included in the term) can be seen as a fairly gradual one and there are a range of

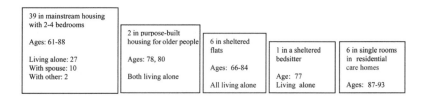

Figure 5.1 Respondents living in housing types, by age range, and whether living alone, with spouse or with other persons(s)

alternative housing forms in the UK that currently accommodate older people (Peace and Holland, 2001). This is not to say, of course, that people always move across this gradient smoothly from one form of accommodation to the next or in one direction only, and people may find themselves making abrupt changes at any time of life. Neither is it true to say that older people invariably see a seamless gradient. Many of the people we interviewed appeared to envisage a qualitative shift between mainstream housing and 'special' environments for older people. Although their understanding of where the limits of the mainstream lay differed depending on how they looked on sheltered housing and their knowledge of it, we have drawn a line for this chapter between mainstream housing and accommodation especially designed with older people in view. Some respondents, however, thought that sheltered housing was a reasonable option for a possible future time when they might want to move into smaller scale accommodation that still allowed more or less independent living. Most said that they would still prefer to stay in their present home for as long as possible, but others saw sheltered housing as a possible bridge between the mainstream housing settings they presently occupied and the very different and special settings represented by the residential home. Several respondents remained unclear about the differences between sheltered housing and residential care homes; for example:

> If I knew that I couldn't cope, you know if I couldn't walk about or couldn't do my own cooking, then yes I think because I have always been very independent I would sell this and go into sheltered housing myself. But I can't, at the moment see that happening, I mean it might I mean I don't know, none of us know what is ahead. But unless I became so that I was conscious that I couldn't cope for myself, then I think I would leave it then until the crisis came. (Belinda)

This respondent also articulates a common resistance to planning for 'dependency', partly on the grounds of the unknowable future, partly from an idea as to how the mainstream and special setting might be differently arranged and ultimately impose a persona they would not wish to assume. From the viewpoint of an older person, living an engaged life in their own home and a familiar community, the person they would become, living an institutionalized life, is unrecognizable.

We would argue that the special setting is best understood if it is contextualized in terms of the mainstream. This is the perspective from which it is viewed by those it is intended to serve and by providers. The analogy of the ordinary domestic home (as in 'homely' or 'a home for life') is frequently invoked by those living and working in the special residential settings to justify prevailing arrangements, although it has to be said that the metaphor of home can be unconvincing when applied to some residential settings and our respondents clearly made a distinction. This was between settings that permitted degrees of 'domesticity' and those that were more forthrightly seen as institutional (nursing homes, hospices and hospitals).

In this chapter, we consider the mainstream setting and argue that it holds features that permit older people to be the selves they wish to be. Our analysis leads us to generalize that this means being able to present themselves to others as complex people with multiple interests and concerns, rather than frail elders whose lives are lived out within spaces and conforming to routines that have been organized by others.

Everyday settings: normative/acceptable/ recognizable

As any number of writers have noted, the mainstream domestic form is a culturally recognizable one (Hillier and Hanson, 1984). Importantly, the house or dwelling is conceived as a 'technical and cognitive instrument, a tool for thought as well as a technology of shelter' (Wilson, 1988, quoted in Birdwell-Pheasant and Lawrence-Zúñiga, 1999, p.4). In other words, the form a dwelling takes, and this would include the disposition of the objects it contains, signifies what is appropriate behaviour by accommodating ordinary, daily enactments and reinforcing custom – a point made by Bourdieu (1977). While we observe great variety in house form and especially in the way the home can be arranged and decorated, forceful arguments have been put forward that the configuration of the spaces that typically make up the home are determined by underlying socio-spatial principles. As we have already suggested, these have to do with the 'public' and the 'private' and associated issues of access, permission and control (Hillier and Hanson, 1984, p.261). They also pivot around appropriateness; for instance, the right activity in the right space, as well as style and fashion. Goffman's (1959) notions of presentation on front or back stage as noted in Chapter 4 are systematized in Hanson and Hillier's mapping of the depth or distance of intimate spaces from the threshold. Rapoport (1969) makes reference to people's ideas of 'the ideal life' in discussing the particular form and spatial configurations that the house assumes in different cultures. This 'ideal life' entails activity systems as well as less functional considerations. Once translated into the domestic form of the house and home, the ideal life is simultaneously instrumental and expressive, material and social, individual and collective. In other words, the homes in which our respondents now lived and to which they referred, as well as the homes they recalled from earlier years, arise out of 'the collective agency' of self and others, including those who are not co-resident – and who may indeed be long gone. Furthermore, we would contend that the notion of the ideal life informs people's own assessments of whether or not they are living a life of quality.

Individuals acting on the materiality of spaces

The material manifestation of all that we understand by the term 'home' produces spaces that contain chosen objects and are configured in such a way as to support daily life for the household as individual, couple or group. Elsewhere (Kellaher et al., 2004) we have argued that it is the aggregate of a lifetime's strategies, in response to the recognition of possibilities and options, that make for a life of quality. In so arguing we suggest that the 'quality of life' that arises as a consequence of external conditions and may be improved by attention to these conditions is only part of the story. It may be that across the life course the balance shifts between the person and constraining external influences – these generally being perceived and experienced as less constraining in earlier years. The research for 'Environment and Identity' reveals older people making highly strategic decisions and moves as they recognize new options in their environments and changing needs in themselves. This is not to say that cultural and normative influences are irrelevant. We have already noted in the opening chapters that the habitus identified by Bourdieu is one expression of a society's culture and norms. The domestic form is culturally variable, which is to say that beyond the broadly cultural domain the domestic form is also gendered and often taken as indi-cative of status or socioeconomic class. The people who have provided the information for this study showed how important it was for them to be living in spaces configured in culturally acceptable ways. This is an issue we follow through here and one that is thrown into sharper relief as we discuss the special settings of sheltered and residential accommodation in the next chapter.

Many would also argue that the home is expressive of stages passed and reached in the life course (Cooper Marcus, 1995; Hockey and James, 2003). This should not surprise us if we accept the obvious fact that the dwelling has the role of supporting daily living for its occu-pants and that as people's capacities and dispositions change, so will the house. Our data suggest that arrangements within the house can also be made to anticipate future points in the life course as the scene is gradually prepared for different circumstances, not least of health and mobility. As we have already discussed with respect to moving house (Chapter 2), not all older people consciously adopt such anticipatory strategies, some preferring to take things as they come and some positively aiming to avoid change in so far as they can.

The house space and the home place it frames and contains also say something about the epoch in which a building was designed and constructed; and indeed about the cohort(s) to which its residents belong. Some of our respondents discussed their own tastes and whether or not they liked to change things; and several also referred to how their tastes and preferences interacted with those of significant others, particularly with spouses, and this sometimes included deceased spouses. For example, this respondent, in his late eighties, was still dealing with rearrangements following the death of his wife 18 months earlier:

> And she was always collecting and hoarding stuff because she might need it some time or other, and we haven't got it all sorted out yet. No, she does. She has really left me with a number of problems of stuff to get rid of, because she had all her mother's stuff, she always said something might be needed some time. (Barry)

Whether we accept the line that older people, because of their invisibility in society, retreat to their home territories to find self-actualization in its relatively uncontested spaces (Mowl et al., 2000) it seems very likely from our data that older people take a lot of pleasure in and maintain confidence levels through the continued power they have to create, alter and adapt the fine details and routines of domestic daily living. Even for those who have become very frail and sometimes immobile, arranging and rearranging small objects and ornaments is important because it demonstrates the importance of agency that can be seriously eroded when others take over tasks that can still be managed. This particularly applies to respondents living in rooms in residential care homes and we go on in Chapter 6 to discuss the effect of these limited spaces on residents' agency.

In this chapter, we review the overall patterning of the spaces in mainstream housing, at the point on the spectrum where the majority of our 54 informants lived. We look at the ways these 39 people arranged the spatial scene for daily living and how they reported on their routinely managed time within the internal domestic spaces and places they used. Physical space is examined first in its extent and internal configuration. We also take into account the way the internal domestic space is positioned in relation to other dwellings and to the neighbourhood discussed in the preceding chapters.

The physical and material aspects of the 54 dwellings in which our informants lived at this point in their varied housing histories could be seen simply as a backdrop to the activities that make daily life – sleeping, washing, cooking, eating and relaxing to name just some of these. Our data reveal, however, what others have argued: that the home space and the objects it accommodates represent much more than a frame for daily living. The idea that the routine minutiae of activities situated within the home space have significance beyond their instrumental value is common to the schema developed by authors discussed in the opening chapter. Rowles, for example, argues for three levels beyond that of the practical and instrumental, showing how routine becomes amplified by emotions and imagination so that the routine domestic is expanded across space and time. This notion of expansion or amplification is an important one to which we return later. Along with Rubenstein and Parmelee, Rowles proposes that the mundane and instrumental activities that sustain daily living also serve to connect the individual to reference groups that lie outside and beyond the home space. In so far as their actions are timely and culturally correct, the individual assumes and is granted a place in the wider scheme of things – in society. This may be demonstrated, for example, in the timing of meals taken alone; so that even those respondents who rose early with an early morning cup of tea, tended to take breakfast later at a 'breakfast time' they consider 'proper' with the radio on or a newspaper to read – thus connecting with the rhythm of the world of work. By the same token, the idea of 'being put to bed at teatime' by carers was anathema to them. The culturally 'correct' rhythm of the day is reflected in the routines described by many of the respondents and discussed in more detail later.

We might make the case that timeliness and correctness rest as much on the capacity of the setting as on the evaluations and subsequent actions of individuals; and that people, perhaps especially in later years, aim to locate themselves in home spaces where they can experience the best and culturally appropriate fit between the intimate aspects of Rubenstein's category of body-centred processes and the larger scale aspects of the built environment. This calculation may go some way to explain why, in spite of their earlier reluctance, many older people actually do arrive at a decision to move into sheltered housing where the scale and convenience of the setting permits such daily situating of self, well before the 'crisis' that they thought would force them to give up their 'own' home.

The 54 dwellings: space occupancy

Approaching one-third of our 54 respondents lived in flats, although these were concentrated in Haringey, where there is a higher than average proportion of flats in sheltered housing, and to a lesser extent in Bedford. Respondents in more rural Northamptonshire tended to live in houses and bungalows. In all three areas, people living in houses tended to have three bedrooms, although one-bedroomed accommodation, often ground floor and with the benefit of gardens, was also found among those in mainstream dwellings. In part, fewer bedrooms reflect age-related housing, particularly sheltered housing provided by the local authority or a registered social landlord. Overall, again one-third of the older people we interviewed had dwellings with at least three bedrooms and two people had four bedrooms. Interestingly, these larger houses both happened to be in Haringey and represent part of the owner-occupied segments of a borough of great contrasts.

As with the informants in a parallel EPSRC study (Hanson et al., 2001), the older people in our study rarely suggested that they had more space than they wanted or could manage. In fact, the reverse was often true and respondents had a whole range of uses for such extra space that, in common with routines and mundane activities, continued to connect them to social networks and to society more generally. For example, several respondents used rooms for hobbies and other activities (office space; photography; sewing) and to accommodate or entertain other people. Even if they were not often used, people in mainstream housing maintain spaces and furniture in spare bedrooms, dining rooms or distinct dining areas. Often people may change the full dining room suite – acquired at marriage perhaps – for a folding or drop-leaf table and just a few of the dining chairs. The activity of making family lunch may be abandoned in its fullest sense, but an important remnant is retained for certain occasions. Extra space in mainstream housing was also used as storage space for their own unused items but also for furniture and possessions belonging to adult children who might be on the move, perhaps between homes or relationships. It also allowed married couples to avoid the stresses of having to share bedroom space when one of them became ill and likely to disturb the other. As one married respondent put it, they had:

> Three nice bedrooms, well two are quite large, one's got a shower in it and a sink. The other one ... the main ... I sleep in one, my wife sleeps in the other because once I had this trouble with this thing I used to have to get up three or four times a night and disturbed her. So I've got used to sleeping in me own double-bed, she sleeps in her own double-bed and that's it, we're quite happy you know. We have a cup of coffee in bed together in the morning and that's it. No problem. (Henry)

The notion that older people require and desire reduced living space has been common among planners. Technically, under-occupation is defined as when a household lives in 'a dwelling which exceeds the bedroom standard by two or more bedrooms' (EHCS, 1998, p.101). This definition allows for the concept of a 'spare' room; the 'bedroom standard' states that 'a separate bedroom is allocated to each cohabiting couple, any other person aged 21 or over, each pair of young persons aged 10–20 of the same sex and each pair of children under 10 regardless of sex' (EHCS, 1998, p.94). It is quite normal for design guidance to make assumptions about the amount of space that different age groups require; for example, guidance for the design of single people's accommodation recommends that young single people should have a minimum floor area of 25 sq. metres, while more mature, middle-aged single adults require at least 32.5 sq. metres (Housing Single People, DOE, 1975). The English Housing Condition Survey (1998) notes that the average floor area for a dwelling in England is around 80 sq. metres. But the range is considerable, with houses constructed before the middle of the 19th century having nearly double the average floor area. Thereafter, the range is reduced towards 70 sq. metres as the post-1990 period of construction is approached. Within this pattern however, housing *type* accounts for more variation; detached houses, unsurprisingly, average 120 sq. metres. Semi-detached houses average 76 sq. metres with terraced houses nearly the same. It is likely that bungalows are included within these three main types as no separate figure is given for them. Some single-storey bungalows are in the form of terraces; but bungalows more often are detached or semi-detached. Flats have around 62 sq. metres where these are in older converted houses. Purpose-built flats, as noted earlier, are more economical of space, averaging 56 sq. metres.

The idea of under-occupation or of reducing living space to something 'manageable' is not, however, as frequently voiced by older people themselves as these policy and practice assumptions might suggest. Indeed, some of our respondents wanted bigger, if not more spaces, especially those who had 'offices' where they maintained computers and linked with the internet. The amount of space in the home and how it is put together are critical factors that can influence the way a person manages and experiences the space and life within it.

Evidence has emerged from a number of studies (Hanson et al., 2001) that clear differences exist between the ways in which most ordinary UK mainstream homes of all types and tenures organize the domestic interior and the ways in which purpose-built older people's housing is typically configured. These differences relate both to the disposition of the main daytime living functions – cooking, dining and living – and also to how bathing and sleeping fit into the overall interior plan. These arrangements embody distinctive approaches to home life that relate to assumptions about age – and have implications for identity construction and its maintenance over time. This is not least in relation to cultural norms about appropriate space for daily living and socializing. It also relates to the juxtaposition of spaces with or without buffer zones offered through circulation space. Kellaher (2002) has shown how circulation space is reduced in purpose-built, often special and age-related, housing.

Because much of the circulation space in houses is provided by staircases, bungalows have reduced circulation areas relative to other dwelling types and small terrace houses have a similar level of habitable space to purpose-built flats. It is significant to note how many of our respondents favoured the bungalow: 'I like bungalows for the fact you don't have any stairs to fall down or fall off, when you get older and you are not so steady on your pins' (Neil).

The mainstream bungalow, with its reduced circulation space and absence of stairs, and perhaps of the gradient changes that make the mainstream dwelling hazardous if mobility fails to any significant degree, nonetheless permits an appropriate level of privacy and acoustic separation. The mainstream terrace house is likely to have similar properties with staircase and separation of levels. Circulation space (including staircase areas) permits passage and separates internal spaces. This both defines spaces according to cultural norms and engenders conditions for more or less visual and acoustic privacy. Within these internal boundaries individuals seek to exercise appropriate degrees of control. This may entail tidiness and the ordering of activities as well as decorative and stylistic preferences. Importantly, the spaces can be organized to maximize the environmental fit already mentioned. The mainstream domestic dwellings that are the focus of this chapter thus appear to permit high levels or privacy and personalization. It is arguable that not all dwelling forms allow the same levels of self-containment or privacy and control. These are important if not crucial, because they allow people to act in ways that tell them that they have variety in their daily lives. The small acts that make up daily living can, as it were, assume an expansive and amplified character unhindered by other people's wishes and actions. In this way, as we shall discuss, identity is practised and constantly adjusted.

The way that individuals fit themselves within the domestic scheme of things varies enormously. On the one hand, there are those who admit that moving house is not a wrench at all: 'Because I have moved so many times in my life' (Bob); on the other hand, there are those who

are entirely centred in their home: 'My home means everything to me
... but the energy is going away from me' (Helen). Only a minority of
our respondents spoke unprompted about the furniture and objects in
their homes in ways that indicated these were important as cues to
memories of those now absent or distant and of earlier days. Most
respondents alluded only very indirectly to the way the home and its
contents evoked other people, places and times. Although we discussed
the past with them, distant past was often related to other places and
recent past to events and people; discussions about the present home
were more likely to focus on current routines within and beyond the
mainstream home and on security and neighbourhood issues. Where
people talked about their past, especially the houses that they had lived
in since childhood, they were less concerned to detail the spatialities of
remembered places than to make the point, albeit indirectly, that they
had complex background; that their present status had been achieved
and accumulated through this passage through particular houses,
streets, neighbourhoods and accompanied variously by constellations
of people; families of origin, friends, colleagues and new families.

While respondents enjoyed the opportunity to describe their past, it
was generally difficult to draw them to be specific about past houses
and their spaces. The point that we want to make here is that the
mainstream dwelling, which is to say the house that has been designed
and built with an 'ordinary' rather than an age-specific population in
view, appears to offer scope for thinking about and explaining oneself
as complex, faceted, creative, resourceful, adaptive and respectably
appropriate – even where eccentricity is claimed. We would also argue
that the mainstream dwelling is spatially configured to contain a varied
and extensive set of objects that the single occupant or couple can use
or contemplate as an integral part of daily living.

Our data, somewhat paradoxically, suggest that it is this very fragmentation or faceting of the materiality of daily life in the mainstream
home that draws the occupant towards action to order and organize
the fragments or components. Through this routine and unavoidable
practice, we suggest that individuals constantly exercise their power to
integrate elements of environment that habitually are or become dispersed. We see this in the way these houses are organized, we hear it in
what people say about their routines and we start to understand that
their objective is to realize in the present moment the biographical

complexities that precede and buttress the experienced older individual. The ultimate rationale for recognizing and then demonstrating such complexity is, we suggest, to justify engagement with others. In Chapter 6 we will reinforce this thesis with reference to special settings. Here, we go on to consider how people apply themselves to the work of integration, in particular through mundane routines.

From instrumental to emotional and imaginative significance of home

For every one of these 39 people the mainstream home had the minimal practical functions of accommodating them and providing a base for their journeys out and about, in and beyond the neighbourhood as discussed in earlier chapters. Harold gives a very clear view of home as a base when he says: 'The house is somewhere to be – you have to live in something . . . but it doesn't mean that much.' This man kept an ordered one-bedroom flat and enjoyed his garden; but most of all he liked to get out and see his friends. The bus route immediately outside was a bonus in this respect. He also said: 'Home is where you live – make friends.' It was clear to him that without this base, friendships would be harder to maintain. Without this base or anchor, the outward-looking perspective that characterized him and many, although not all, of the men to whom we talked would be less meaningful. This is in spite of this strong orientation to the outdoors and neighbourhood. While his domestic scene was fairly minimal with little decorative ornamentation within the flat, it contained objects that he could draw on to explain who he was and where he was from. A family photograph showing him as a young child, along with three generations of family, was displayed relatively prominently and discussed in detail with recollective elaboration and some animation. Similarly, his considerable CD collection was pointed out and could have been the focus of an extended account of his tastes and preferences over the years. In no sense can it be said that these items were 'on display' as if to advertise 'identity'. But, as with the other respondents, he revealed himself as someone who had a range of connections and interests. Of course, we could also say that his strategies served to conceal as well as reveal.

With this group of older people at least, furniture and objects – large and small – were only rarely indicated as important. Nearly all the objects in most of the respondents' homes needed to be decoded by them for any significance to be revealed to others:

> I don't have too much difficulty over that, that is the only photo I have got of my husband. I had those frames for my ... that frame, and those ones and the one my daughter is in ... that was bought for my 25th wedding anniversary. When my husband died I thought I have got to have something, somewhere, and that is an old one, and it is the only one I have got where he is on his own. And that was taken in Majorca by a friend. So I stuck that in there. And then I came across this snap of him and I put it in that frame. And my daughter had a number of photographs taken and I liked that one, so that is why that one is in there. And that is the only photograph of my son because he won't have a photograph taken, and he has got two degrees and do you think he would go and get either of them so I could have a photograph taken? No. So I had to find one so I could stick it in that frame. That was taken by the same person who took that one, and I did have one of my daughter as well. But he is only about 17 there. And this of course is a graduation photograph. So that is the only reason I have got them in ... oh, my sister framed that one of my parents' wedding and gave it to me for some Christmas or something. And she gave me that one of me and my mother again for my silver wedding, or something like that. So they are not ones I have thought anything specially ... I am waiting for a wedding photograph or something, but they don't produce those. (Naomi)

In other words, while Harold appeared to live a pared-down domestic life, his situation was not so different to others like Naomi who spent more time and gave more attention to their homes. It may be the case that the expectation that objects – almost as fetishes – will feature as central to identity in later years has arisen in relation to the multitude of studies that have looked at special rather than mainstream domestic settings. As we will see in the following chapter the 'editing' required when a residential move is to be made, to accommodate the material items accumulated over several decades, generally in family situations, seems to lead, as the social sedimentation or clutter in which materialities have been embedded becomes cleared away, to the exposure of objects themselves.

In her late sixties, Helen is one of the younger respondents and lives with several family members. She appears to think of herself as still more or less central within her family and social network. The power of the setting to influence mood or general disposition is revealed by Helen when she says: 'This house – it makes me feel happy. It is the centre of everything.' She refers to the way the large family house, described as 'well maintained, with double glazing and central heating' allows three generations to cohabit, as individuals need to be accommodated from time to time. While she describes the house as the centre of everything, her accounts of the comings and goings of her grown-up children and of her grandchildren, her management of the logistics entailed – who goes in which room, and the shopping and mealtime arrangements – also indicates how she is just as central to the extended family and to seeing that their needs are met. In this instance, and in most others, the mainstream home is frame, context and vehicle for individuals who invariably aim to place themselves as close as possible to their significant networks; a finding that also emerged as central in the EPSRC study, *From Domesticity to Care* (Hanson, 2003).

Where such networks are less strong, as with Betty, who recounts a long working life as live-in housekeeper with few family connections, it seems that the materialities of home life, the furniture and the objects, may be acknowledged more explicitly as significant: 'This is all my own furniture. I should hate to be put in some place where all the furniture is provided, or it is a furnished place. Here I can do what I like and when I like – no ties at all.' Living in a one-bedroom flat provided by a housing trust, Betty seems to be alert to the realities of living in other people's territory. Her working life as a housekeeper entailed responsibilities and, through these, connections with others, even though her access to and control of personal space was necessarily restricted. It seems that in her assessment her social roles offset the personal restrictions. With retirement however, the social roles fell away, bringing into focus the need to establish a territory for a future social identity to be established. She speaks, however, of wanting to maintain firm boundaries: 'My own kitchen? Very important; I would hate to be tied up with somebody else.'

Not everyone who moves to special/sheltered housing sets such tight boundaries, and certainly not in defensive ways, even where as with Brenda, this has meant the switch from a large family house and responsibility for husband and eight children, to a bedsitter. She also 'likes the freedom ... I don't have to ask anybody'. She considers whether or not she would want to be closer to one or more of her grown children and concludes that, being confident of her secure place within the family's affections, she chooses to remain near friends. She speaks of her limited mobility and exhausted reserves of strength: 'I can't do [things] now. I have to live on memories a lot and says: "I had my go".' Although these instances do not involve mainstream housing, they are cited here because they show how the social overrides the material. In other words, the environment is certainly crucial but people suggest that it is crucial because it serves the purpose of making and sustaining important social connections.

Home was also an important place for the male informants, but many of them described lives where their routines took them outside their homes, so that the dwelling seemed to be a home base. Ben, for instance, says that: 'Home, means staying indoors, routines, feeling secure.' He makes no reference at all to the spaces of his home or to the furnishings. Like Harold, described earlier, Ben also stresses the importance to him of music, and adds 'not things'. This interview is remarkable for the level of introspection that dominates his comments and responses. He reflects on past relationships that have not always gone smoothly and follows up with speculation and introspection as to why this might have been the case. He tends not to discuss the physical or material features of his homes, except in response to direct questions.

As already suggested, this is not just a characteristic of the men in this study. While widows and couples could all point to favourite items and say why they would be protected and transported to a new home (a mix of history and significant people, such as children and grandchildren), most informants only did this when specifically asked to focus on such memories and associations. Most of the time, in describing their lives and the environment from which and in which they created and enacted the roles that generated identity, people spoke of the spatial patternings that their daily routines established through temporal ordering.

Routines

The effect of adopting routines is to temporalize space. Routines do not take place as mental exercises, although a lot of thought does go into establishing regular arrangements as people optimize their own energy. People also take opportunities to integrate with the routines of other people both inside their own home and in other places. For our sample, anyway, routines seem to establish an order that defines boundaries of space, for instance, between individuals in couples and routines also construct an ordered trajectory along which daily life progresses with some semblance of control. That control over time is, in the long term, illusory may make the construction and following of routines more important in later life than in earlier years. While the disruption of routines could be welcomed on occasions, for example, when being taken out for a birthday treat, on the whole disruptions tended to be regarded as a nuisance because they would involve the reordering of activities that otherwise did not demand much thought or organization. This habitual state of affairs seemed to arise after retirement when time was available to organize and a strong impulse to order things and time seemed to arise. For most, adult children were by then established in other households. But, for a few, capacity to order things might be reduced where they were asked to store furniture and possessions and sometimes to accommodate an adult child who was temporarily without a base of their own. This preference for routine was discussed in one of the focus groups and one participant described how she took part in occasional family outings to keep her family happy and unworried about her, even though she actually preferred her usual routine.

Many descriptions of people's routines incorporate some seasonality in the frequency of going out and staying indoors as the length of day and weather conditions vary. As we have described in Chapter 3, most respondents were protective of themselves in terms of potential harm outdoors at particular times – especially in the dark or when the pavements were slippery. Marking the passage of time by planning for and acknowledging significant dates was an essential part of our respondents' demonstration of who they were, whether these were cultural events such as Christmas; personal anniversaries; or the turning of the seasons. Seasons were marked by such annual routines as getting out the winter coats; or starting to put out birdseed in spring; or changing the curtains from heavy to light. Some of the respondents described how they had (regretfully) started to pull back from these kinds of activity – for example, they were sending fewer and fewer Christmas cards or had stopped bothering with annual bedding plants. We would suggest that the regret relates perhaps to an unconscious and certainly unspoken acknowledgement of the beginnings of losses to do with having a firm 'grip' on environments.

Most people also made reference to weekdays and weekends in relation to routines: 'We never go out at weekends. But we only stay in once a week!' (Neil). As was the case for many people we talked to, this couple were involved – both separately and together – in several local clubs and organizations. Both of them also had interests and hobbies that they pursued at home. The husband did painting and photography and had a designated space for these activities; the wife was 'attached to her books' and had ordered these in particular parts of the house. Another couple with a similar range of interests that entailed both going out and staying in said of their living room: 'This is a living room – full of things to do – not just a set.'

Everyone in mainstream housing we interviewed described quite complex routines. All appeared to have associative lives they considered satisfying with family and friends who were significantly present either physically or emotionally. However, some of those who lived alone were prepared to admit times of loneliness and these were more likely to be experienced in long winter evenings and at weekends if they did not have family visits at these times. With a more limited range of opportunities for interesting activities then, respondents relied more than ever on routines to 'populate' the hours of being alone. The respondent whose words follow describes the importance to her, after the death of her co-resident sister, of a nightly phone call from a younger friend:

> I think one of the things that have helped me very much to adapt is ...
> having this very good friend and she rings me up every night, somewhere
> between 10–10.30 pm and we always have a good laugh or a good chat
> before I go off upstairs. And this is quite a focal point really. Because I
> always know this phone call is coming and that has helped me a lot. And
> I think it is quite fair to say that she hasn't missed more than a dozen
> nights phoning me since my sister died, she has rung up every night, and
> this makes quite a difference to my life. She hasn't got the time to see me,
> she works very, very hard, and very long hours but she does phone me
> every night. It ends my day; that is right. I hear everything she has done,
> she wants to know what I have done. When I was ill she kept in very close
> touch with me. This made a lot of difference to me. (Hannah)

As we have described in Chapter 3, many respondents were involved with local organizations and offered help to other people. Many were involved in reciprocal relationships that gave them either practical support or the sense that there were people around who would help when necessary. Even those who made comments such as 'Nothing routine about me!' went on to illustrate an ordered pattern of movement within the home. The importance of 'doing what I like when I feel like it' was also stressed, though more by those who lived on their own than those living with others.

Importantly, however, routines require the kind of space and spatial boundaries that are culturally accepted as constituting the normative domestic dwelling. Whether people described themselves as highly routinized or more casual in their routines, they operated within and between the spaces of the home. There was a constant refrain of the adjustment of spaces to accommodate changing patterns of the household and activities in the home spaces. Some people had adapted their homes, like the couple who had occupied the same dormer bungalow for decades, adding and changing the arrangement of bedrooms as the family increased and then declined. Now, as they age, the husband was able to say: 'While there is two of us I can envisage coping because we have got everything on the ground floor.'

Others had made adjustments by moving. One family had moved between bungalows in the same area. These relocations, while apparently not dissimilar, had subtle differences; increasingly with each move the garden space had become smaller and the number of bedrooms reduced from four to three to two (Nicholas). Manageability of house and garden and the need to release equity from the larger houses of earlier years had guided the moves this couple had made, with a detailed insider knowledge of the neighbourhood, over the previous 20 years. Along with these considerations was their unwavering determination to stay in an area where they had many contacts and were well established, and in which their routine associations could maintain an unbroken pattern of place-congruent continuity (Twigger-Ross and Uzzell, 1996).

The paradox we uncover here is that while one of the defining characteristics of home for many of our respondents was the sense that you can do what you like, when you like (i.e. act out of routine), what they actually did in creating the home space was to *protect* their own routines. We would argue that for older people living in mainstream housing, routines act as temporal anchor points through which the ordering we have already proposed for spatial and material aspects of environment can take place. Thus, the need to order space and time within the environment allows the individual to practise and rehearse integrating components of environment. Through this habitual activity, we argue, an integrated and coherent identity is produced. Furthermore, we make the case that this is the sine qua non for social interaction, a cognitive anchor point. As we go on to discuss in Chapter 6, the routines followed by residents in care homes are not of the same order because they are so heavily dictated by others both temporally and spatially, so that an individual's routinization becomes concentrated on more accessible objects and perhaps the internal life of the mind.

Conclusion

The focus of this chapter has been on the way older people act within and on the internal spaces of the ordinary domestic dwelling so that it is experienced as a secure base for daily activity and, out of this, for identity construction and maintenance. The analysis of data collected from our respondents leads us to support the claim that people derive the security and confidence to use and enjoy their material and social surroundings only when they have a secure starting point. The notion of the home as an anchor point from which to venture forth into the neighbourhood and wider community has emerged in previous chapters. Evidence from other studies tends to support this analysis. For example, in our study of residential homes in the 1980s (Wilcocks et al., 1987) we found that the residents who acted in more outgoing ways were those who had a room of their own. This group were much more likely to say that they had made friends and that they were less homesick than was the case for the residents who had to share a room – generally with a stranger.

Notions of environment and identity hint at the conceived, perceived and the lived worlds, both inner and external, that are implied in daily life (Lefebvre, 1991). The interaction of these worlds is crucial to understanding how people make their homes work for them and the sense of self they aim to secure. We have noted elsewhere (Kellaher et al., 2004) that the fixed items and domains that underpinned earlier quality-of-life studies become secondary to the more dynamic mechanism or sets of strategies that older individuals bring into play as they keep themselves going and, although few actually used such terms, make a life of quality. Through these informants' accounts of their neighbourhoods, their homes and the lives and expectations they build there, the trajectories or pathways linking the inner and external worlds begin to come into focus. Broadly, the accounts show how people try to manoeuvre themselves into positions that are physically and socially comfortable and maximize their influence over the material and the social. They do this within their networks, however fragile these may have become with the accumulation of changes and the build-up of uncertainty with age and over time.

While older people have specific needs for space to accommodate their daily routines, leisure, social potency – and, conversely, their privacy – this need for space does not seem to be adequately provided for in the actual housing that many older people occupy, certainly in 'special' accommodation, but also in much mainstream housing.

Yet older people themselves do recognize their need for sufficient space; many of the participants in the EPSRC study (Hanson et al., 2001) for example expressed the view that the 'right' amount of space for older people was a home that has two public rooms and two bedrooms. The minimum is, perhaps, a home with three habitable rooms that can be used interchangeably to allow for flexibility and choice in later life, in addition to the kitchen and bathroom.

At the other end of the spectrum of space provision, flats with just a bed-sitting room tend to be among the most inflexible of all when it comes to accommodating variety within older people's lifestyles. The number and type of physical fixes in this type of living space mean that it is usually difficult to use in ways other than as dictated by its designed intention. The current generation of older people are already showing a much greater awareness of the limitations of this type of accommodation than did the previous generation of elders for whom sheltered housing of this type was originally built and antipathy to it is likely to increase for each subsequent group of elders. Certainly among our respondents, this kind of accommodation was totally unacceptable whether or not they thought it possible they themselves might move into sheltered housing; and indeed several respondents thought that one-bedroomed flats were also too small.

In this chapter, we have argued that the temporal patternings represented by daily routines, enacted spatially within the home in ways which take account of anchor points and their wider domestic contexts, are the constituent parts from which environmental identity is constructed. In the next chapter, we go on to examine how these crucial elements relate to environments that have been created for older people by virtue of their age.

6

Pacing the self

Introduction

We have seen in the preceding chapter how, at the stage in the life course when most of our informants continued to live in ordinary, mainstream domestic environments, daily life is most likely to be structured by routines that we have termed temporal markers, in contrast to spatialities. It is thus, through movement within a local social milieu as well as in and out of the local and domestic environment, that sense of self and the identity that arises with it, is established and maintained. In other words, the domestic routines people have established over time mesh with the multiple outside contacts and commitments taken on with retirement, to underpin identity as it is revealed through time. These crucial routine associations could not, of course, be recognized as such if they were not enacted in a familiar place, so spatial structures clearly come into play. However, at the stage in life and in housing history that we have discussed in relation to living in mainstream homes, temporal rather than spatial structures seemed to predominate in shaping people's accounts of their experiences of environment inside and beyond the mainstream home.

In this chapter, we look at the 15 people who were living in housing especially designed for older people (see Figure 5.1) rather than in mainstream housing. We take further the arguments made in the preceding chapter. Principally, we examine how what is viewed as a qualitative shift in environmental circumstances is actually experienced and we consider how any contrasts our respondents reveal can help us to understand the impact of environment on identity. Of the 15 people in these special environments, six were living in single rooms in residential care homes when we interviewed them. The others lived in housing types distributed along a continuum ranging from purpose-built flats containing two bedrooms to a sheltered bedsitter that had a kitchenette and en suite bathroom. We can see that each of these dwellings has the basic 'ingredients' of housing – sleeping space, living space and bathing/toileting space. Food preparation space is absent in the individual residential settings. While it is valid to say there is a gradient between the mainstream and the special commented on in Chapter Five, we have to ask at what point is a move experienced as a qualitative shift and why should this be?

Focusing on the transition between mainstream and special environments, we argue in this chapter that the move into accommodation designed and built with an older and frailer group in mind seems to be accompanied in the main by a switch in the individual's focus from the predominantly temporal structures associated with routine associational life to the spatial structures of the interior of the dwelling. Where the pared-down interiors and routines of the residential home are concerned and where personal dwelling arrangements are contained within a single space, the focus often comes to rest on micro-level interactions such as with the arrangement of objects therein – photographs and memorabilia displayed with special care; clothes and other belongings ordered within the confined space available.

In other words, agency and intentions that may have to do with the maintenance of identity are likely to be transferred to the material confines of environment, as routine and associations become reduced or restricted. We make the case for a connection between reduced associational life and pared-down environment and we consider the extent to which there may be a causal link. It is true that the proportion of the informants in this study who lived in residential care is very small. However, the reader can also draw on the observations made by the very many older people studied in research (by ourselves and others) on residential care. The speculations of our respondents in mainstream housing who viewed the prospect of such moves from – they hoped – a distance are also important here, even though they may not be borne out by actual experience.

What emerges in discussion about the concepts and meanings of home with individuals and couples who continue to live in terraced houses, detached and semi-detached houses, bungalows and flats –

even where the last may be purpose built for older people – is a level of apprehension about having to move into certain forms of special housing. In these instances, people were generally referring to residential homes and often nursing homes would be subsumed within this label or within the general term 'old people's homes'; and as we have seen sometimes respondents were also referring to special housing such as sheltered housing of various kinds. Here, we first consider residential care as being at the extreme point of the domestic continuum and then look at the sheltered accommodation that people in mainstream housing regarded as either an alternative to or a stepping stone towards the higher levels of care and support that might become necessary – if one lived long enough and became frail.

Anticipating specialized accommodation

The majority of our informants who were still living in mainstream housing noted two particular aspects of the residential home scenario as problematic, if not outright negatives: that there was nothing to do all day long and that there was an enforced association with people they might not want to mix with:

> I went to see one of my old work pals, he is in an old folks home. They are just sitting in a room with their backs to the wall. Especially this time of year, I think they provide entertainment. They had a male singer yesterday morning, and a children's class. They do try, but it is a horrible existence, just sitting there. (Bill)

> I don't like that at all. It smells of pee doesn't it? I am very unkind. Yes I have [visited], because there were several people here that went into homes because they needed nursing care, it wasn't just living in a safe place, they were old and they needed nursing care, so. They did their best. Some are better than others, I used to go and see a lady that was in the one just over the hill, on the corner, oh what is it called? . . ., that was rather nice. I think that was . . . you had to pay a bit more for that I think. But that was very nice. But in all of them, they just sit around looking at things or going to sleep, whatever. But there again that is all you want to do I suppose, they don't want to be entertained. (Bonny)

> Yes and they don't have anything of their own, this is another thing that I hated for my mother-in-law, she had an L-shaped room and there was a

person here and she was there in the L-shape, so she actually wasn't ... although she had part of a room to herself, she didn't have a whole room to herself. Whereas my friend's mother, in this Jewish home, she had her own room, she could have her own telephone, she had her own bathroom. You know, and things around her that she could have to herself, and I think old people should be entitled to that sort of thing. And they are not are they? So often they are ... I wouldn't want to be forever with other people, because sometimes you should be free to move from one to the other. I am sure it must be difficult, if you can't walk for instance, to be taken ... I don't know, it does worry me, that does. (Naomi)

The residents mentioned in these observations are spoken of as members of a discrete category. There is little that the speakers seem to regard as common in these residents' lives compared to the lives of the majority of older people among whom they would claim to locate themselves. It may be fair to say that the world being described is an 'unnatural' one – no possessions, shared space and people with whom there is and can be no connection. Thus, people tended to express their anxieties – for they were often thinking about what the coming years might hold for them personally – in terms of no longer having any obvious social or productive role. Speaking frequently, as we see from these quotations, from experiences of visiting family or friends who had moved into residential care, they would also try to counter their critical tone by acknowledging how good the care and kind the staff could be (echoed by those respondents actually living in residential care homes). Respondents spoke of the difficulty of sharing space and being forced into contact with people they did not know. Thus, they refer to spatial characteristics of residential care, but as a vehicle for anxiety about having to mix daily with unfamiliar people; associational life appears to be at issue as well as personal identity when forced into degrees of intimacy:

Yes, I ... I always ... it would worry me to go to an old people's home. I hope I never do, I hope I die before I go into an old people's home. Because I couldn't bear to ... I couldn't sit there you know arguing about whether the windows should be open or closed. I couldn't stand it. (Naomi)

I have been in several old people's homes to visit and again that is another high horse of mine, if I had one I would have individual tables where people could sit around in groups and talk to each other. What I hate about homes, even the better ones, is the fact that they have chairs all around the room and ... unless you can actually talk to your immediate next door neighbour, although you are in the same room, you have no contact. I know not all of them are capable of doing this, but ... I think to live in that type of home you become ... to coin a phrase 'institutionalized'. As I say if I run a home it would be on very different lines, those that are capable I would enable them if you like to sit together and talk to each other and possibly have a little game of cards, which a lot of people my age, I don't play cards, and older do. So as far as I am concerned I am going to say I hope to goodness that I never get to that stage that I have to go into an old people's home. But sheltered housing I would quite happily accept. (Belinda)

Nevertheless, some respondents were aware of closures of local residential homes and issues about funding residential care and even though they did not really want to go into a residential care home, the thought that such a facility might not be available if they needed it was also a worry:

And it is quite frightening actually, because ... I have just been in the hospital and seeing some of the older ... you know in their 80s and 90s and having experienced with my own parents and [husband's] parents you know, how they were and how we looked after them, but they had to go into residential care. Well dad didn't, we looked after him. But my mother and [husband's] mother, they did, and my mother had a type of dementia. And now my last surviving uncle, he has got Alzheimer's, and to see them you think 'that is only 20 years on from us now' you know, and you think 'what is there going to be for us?' especially with all these changes that are happening really. It is a worry. (Nullah)

Respondents who were not living in this kind of accommodation acknowledged that it necessitated some restriction of autonomy. Many, like Belinda, just quoted, could envisage themselves living in sheltered accommodation, even though they preferred to stay where they were, but living in a residential care home was almost unthinkable unless they should become very frail or confused. At the same time, a proportion of informants admitted that the time might well come when such a move would be necessary, although for some this was framed as a decision to be approached incrementally. Sheltered housing could be a preliminary stage through which the move to residential care might (or might not) be contemplated and approached:

Well, the thing is, to me it comes in stages. First I would move to a smaller place, possibly a smaller garden and possibly sheltered housing but that is about as far as I would go ... That's my limit ... If I get taken into a home I'll have to ... or something I am about to you know. As long as I have a brain in my head, and I am able to do things, that's about as far as I go, sheltered housing. But I'm not going any further. (Neil, married, living in mainstream housing)

Both residential care homes and traditional sheltered housing are well established and many people have visited friends and relatives in them. On the whole, our respondents considered the possibility of the latter with more equanimity and a few were actively considering making such a move. Even those who did not think that it would suit them thought that there was a role for sheltered housing:

Sheltered? Excellent, excellent. But of course our standards are so low, I always refer people in this area when they go to Bury St Edmund's to go and have a look at [name]. Now I find that how it should be, excellent. It might not be everybody's choice but I find it excellent, the accommodation is first class, the attention to the detail to suit requirements is first class, its cleanliness and safety aspects, and everybody is welcome there. I find it a very, very pleasant environment, it is built in an area where it is pleasant for people. (Brian)

Yet for a minority of respondents the material, spatial and social circumstances of sheltered housing were considered to be simply inadequate to their aspirations:

Not too keen on them, my dad ended up in one. He ended up living in a little box. I find them claustrophobic. The people here live in places like that and they seem quite happy with them, but I am used to having the space around, I always had the space around me, and to be herded into a little box, especially if I was on my own, I think it would blow my mind. I don't think I would last too long in one of those. I think I would go under very, very quickly. (Bernard)

We will return to the question of spatial allocation in this sample of special housing after we have considered what the six respondents who actually lived in residential care had to say about it.

Living in residential care homes

Now we consider the experiences and observations of those older people in this study who had reached what the others believed was the end of the line and what Townsend (1962) called the 'last refuge'. Six of our informants were living in residential care at the time they talked to us, two men and four women, their ages spanned 87 to 93 years. All but one, who was experiencing a short-stay and had already decided that residential care was not for him, had made what they expected to be a permanent move. Most had done so for health reasons, although one (Nerys) had been settled in a home for a couple of decades having been moved for social and housing reasons in her sixties – a placement that would be unusual now.

It has to be said that of the five 'permanent' residents, four were mostly very content with the settings in which they now found themselves. Although upset by recent bereavements, they did not generally say that they were homesick for the home or the furniture or the neighbourhood they had left behind or that they were spatially over-constrained. This was especially notable with regard to those older women in their later eighties whose health had declined and whose families had both urged and advised them that residential care was the best way forward.

The wish to relieve close family, often adult children already retired themselves, from the worry and responsibility of an aged and now unpredictably frail parent or older relative was categorized as a 'legit-imate' explanation for entering residential care in our first study (Willcocks et al., 1987). In that analysis of 1000 residents, those who settled best into the new home were most likely to be the third that gave such explanations. The older women in focus in this present study, and indeed some of those who had moved into scaled-down special, sheltered housing, spoke as equal collaborators in a plan for the rest of their family. Significantly, however, they had all moved into space that was a fraction of that in which they had previously lived. For the respondents in residential care homes, their bedroom space, although small, represented an acceptable compromise with other considerations: 'Well I can't move about much, so it is [big enough] really. I mean, I couldn't get around the bed without hanging on' (Bronwyn); 'We saw a bigger one, but I wanted one with a bathroom, which is essential for me' (Beryl).

Routines

While three of the care home residents were taken for trips out of the home very regularly by their families, the rest usually stayed in the home for most of the time. Routines within the homes were very much timetabled around meals and getting up and going to bed:

> I usually go down in the morning for breakfast about 7 am, I get up and do everything in my own room and leave it tidy and make my own bed and do all those sorts of things. And I always leave it completely tidy so people don't have to do anything when they go in. And I do that and come down and have breakfast. And we have lunchtime about 12.30 pm and an evening meal about 5 pm. But I usually go to bed about 7 pm from here, sit around and watch the television and then go up to bed at ... no, 9 pm not 7 pm and make my way up the stairs to my own bedroom. But I never stay here until about 11 pm, because by about 9 pm you are getting a little bit tired when you have had all day down here you know. (Herbert)

Bronwyn, after getting up at 8.00 am, usually does:

> Nothing [laughs] I either sit and read or ... maybe watch television or ... I mean, it is surprising how quickly it goes, by the time breakfast is over it is sort of 10 am. And you are going back again for lunch at 12–12.30 pm. And ... they bring a cup of tea around in the afternoon. I am about the last [to go to bed] I think. I do stay up until about 10.00 pm. (Bronwyn)

Aged 93, Bronwyn is very comfortable with this pace of life. These two quotations highlight the differences between residents in the extent to which they remain actively involved in the care of themselves and their environments; some wanting to do as much for themselves as possible: 'I try to do everything myself, while I can' (Beryl). Others enjoying being cared for: 'Well I don't have to think for myself, organizing and everything, it is all done for me. And what they don't do, my daughter does. I couldn't be bothered to do any more' (Bronwyn); 'I like having all the meals cooked for me. Not knowing what you are going to have every day, you know' (Nelly).

This resident is voicing an important point about routines and since we have suggested that routine is one way in which people bring together certain 'dispersed' facets of their day-to-day lives, we need to address this. For many older people a time may arrive where routine practice is no longer routine because previously taken-for-granted actions become the focus for constant deliberation as they have to weigh up the pros and cons – and perils – of, for instance, having a bath or cooking a meal. Constant attention to such minutiae becomes wearing and, we suggest, other options have to be brought into focus. Residential care may be one of these if, as for Bronwyn, they 'cannot be bothered any more'.

However, there are trade-offs that can have a downside. Even though the decision to move into a residential care home might be taken in a supportive family context and the room size and pace of life acceptable in the context of other factors, residents may still experience boredom: 'It is a bit boring in the afternoons. Sometimes Julie, one of the head ones, she does get a quiz up sometimes. And that is good fun. But mostly it is quite boring unless you have got a good book' (Nelly). Or they may feel disempowered by regulations: 'We are not supposed to make our own things here. They don't like people going into the kitchen and taking over things, no' (Harriet). And for many people, having made the difficult decision to move from their own home into a care setting, the adjustment to a different way of life can be very challenging.

Among our sample, Beryl had moved into a home the most recently and we interviewed her a few months afterwards. She had one friend there with whom she regularly took coffee and she spent quite a lot of time outside the home with her daughters. But when she was in, she tended to take meals in her own room and reported that there were few other residents that she could have a conversation with, finding the confusion of many of the residents difficult to cope with: 'My family said when I came "you are to have lunch in the dining room" but one lady is so beyond it that she kept muttering and it made me depressed. So I had them in here. I am sorry, because it gives them more work, and they are so good and so busy.' Beryl felt that she had changed since moving into the home:

> Beryl: Well I used to do jigsaws, play patience, and I went to a toy making club, soft toys. And that kept me busy you know, because I could bring them home and do them. And I love the garden, I used to do bits in the garden.

[*Interviewer*: So what do you do now that you are here?]

Beryl: Do you know, it is a very funny thing, since I have been here I have got lots to do, but I don't want to do it.

[*Interviewer*: Really, that is interesting.]

Beryl: And before I came I used to eat no end of Thornton's toffee, and my grandson gave me that big box for Christmas, and I haven't touched it.

[*Interviewer*: Really?]

Beryl: I have completely altered.

With eye problems, she was also reading much less and watching television much more. Beryl said that she was trying not to dwell on the past because she found it painful, but with time on her hands it was hard not to. Within a relatively short space of time, Beryl had lost her husband and her home and moved in with strangers living a still-alien lifestyle. Despite the convenience and comfort of her room and living near to her attentive daughters, it should not come as a surprise that she would show signs of depression. Arguably the minimization of environmental press had allowed other considerations to make more of an impact on her life and she had not yet had time to adjust to new routines and ways of remaining connected with her considerably altered environment: 'It is very difficult ... it is so different, completely. This room in a way reminds me more of boarding school. But ... I mean they are so kind, you couldn't wish for anybody kinder.'

While this resident, who can still go out of the home regularly, makes a statement about identity and its alteration, it does not seem to have been made in the same despairing tone as those many residents in other studies who have remarked: 'I never thought it would come to this.'

Whether or not they become accustomed to life in a residential care home, older people living in these very specialized settings appear to experience a distinct trade-off between decreased autonomy and more security. Clearly, for some people this is acceptable – either because they relish being taken care of, or for less positive reasons because they feel that they have reached the end of the road. Others regard it as an unfortunate necessity. How this trade-off is put into operation and experienced also depends to a large extent on the regime in the home and the agenda of those running the home and doing the caring. It is these people who manage the rhythm of the day and the kinds of activity and socialization that are possible. While most care home residents seem to cope better in these environments than older people living outside them predict that they themselves would manage, it is clear that opportunities for re-engagement and the range of options open to them may be severely limited. Older people living in main-stream housing appear to recognize and to resist the strong likelihood of becoming 'completely altered'.

Institutionalization is the term used to describe the processes that are likely to bring about such change in the individual (Goffman, 1961). Here we have the chance to consider how far environment contributes to changed identities and how far old age and frailty may be respon-sible. These six people spoke of diminished spaces, routines established by the home, of having to be with unknown people and of being at a loss to know what to do. Other studies (Peace et al., 1997; Kellaher, 2000) have shown how difficult it can be to make new associations and contacts in these settings. One explanation offered is that the cues available in mainstream daily living are absent and their equivalents are unrecognizable – until the institution's code has been learnt and absorbed. And yet, we see here older people, weary from the effort of not managing routine daily life within the mainstream, finding much to appreciate in settings that offer care, support and kindness. We need to examine the trade-off between residential and mainstream daily living in order to question whether it is unavoidable or whether there is middle ground – perhaps represented by extra-care sheltered housing?

We have seen that in mainstream housing it is possible to reveal or conceal aspects of the self and thus to work on identity for oneself and for presentation to others. This is hardly possible in these extremely special settings since frailty and a corresponding support are the two faces of the 'currency' of care. Spatial allocations in residential settings are such that the environment is likely to be a miniaturized one. While there is a lot of variation in what space is provided, the regulatory standard at 12 sq. metres for new build single bedroom and 10 sq. metres for pre-existing homes[1] is such that daily life can be very compressed. Of course, residents are expected to live a convivial life and to move into the public spaces, but not all wish to do so, particularly if they do not find the company such that it supports their idea of themselves or the person they wish to show to their family members or remaining friends who visit. These are just a few of the points at which mainstream and residential life diverge and they are well-known and accepted facts. Do they, in fact, work against the maintenance of identity as people have recognized it in mainstream dwellings?

If the argument we began to develop in Chapter 5 is taken forward with this material on residential living at the opposite end of the spectrum (Figure 5.1) it becomes as follows. In mainstream life, and here we are considering post-retirement years, although it should also hold for earlier phases, identity is sustained through the integrating processes that bring together the fragments of daily life. Achievement of a coherence in one's environment entails having an 'ordered' house and a correspondingly ordered set of associations. The constant practice of ordering spaces, places, objects and of encountering people in or from this setting, we argue is what maintains and adjusts identity. When there is little if anything remaining to bring into coherence, to work on creatively, the identity-practising process must grind to a halt. Perhaps it is displaced and becomes the biographical task of end of life; adjusting to the loss of the other and preparing for the loss of self (Freud, 1917). In such a case, observation and discourse may not give us evidence that a different identity building task is underway.

The point we need to make here, if this argument is to hold up, is that residential care removes the material with which older people can practise identity construction. We know that residential rooms are not tenured in the same way as any mainstream dwelling and the foundation of territoriality may thus be insecure. We know that many things – furniture, clothing, objects, ephemera, must be discarded when such a move is made. It would follow that as concealment of frailty becomes very unlikely, revealing oneself as a complex person with decades of antecedent events 'laid down' as the base of identity, also becomes very difficult. Life is lived in a unicellular setting, associations are reduced for many reasons and activity that links an individual with life and people beyond the home is infrequent. There is little left to order and we argue it is the paucity of space, objects and routines that leads to identity becoming more fixed than dynamic. In this sense, environment can be said to inhibit the production and reproduction of identity.

Having made such a bold claim, we need to consider what happens when we focus on sheltered housing. This has been designed with older people in mind, although it has a fuller complement of familiar environmental cues than is the case for the very unusual residential setting.

Living in sheltered housing

The life of respondents living in sheltered housing differed from that of the people in residential care homes in some fundamental ways. In all, six respondents lived in sheltered housing and two in accommodation for older people without a resident warden (of the type of housing previously known as 'part one' accommodation). In these settings they had more personal space; they had autonomy over the rhythm of their day; and they could come and go from home more independently. Their curatorial role within their living space was greater and more complex, and they retained responsibility for more aspects of their daily life including shopping, cooking and cleaning. Relative to respondents living in mainstream housing, they had ceded some responsibilities, which typically included maintaining space within their home for other people; looking after the 'family home' and its contents; maintenance and gardening; and for some the responsibilities of home ownership. There was also a tendency for their social life to become increasingly focused within the sheltered housing scheme itself rather than in the wider community, particularly if they had mobility problems. Nevertheless, for most of them, the sheltered housing flat or bungalow was more meaningfully their own home, because it was self-contained. It was not anyone else's territory and privacy could be maintained in spaces that were both intimate and public.

However, it is not always easy for people to make the move to sheltered housing, and Hermoine describes the process by which she eventually took the step after her husband died:

> [T]he family wanted to know what I was going to do ... and I said I would start applying for a small flat somewhere. And I was just dreading that I would end up in an old people's home, I was just dreading it. And sheltered housing, the very name 'sheltered housing' I didn't even think about.

A social worker took her to view a sheltered flat, close to shops but at the top of a hill:

[T]he hill would have been awe inspiring, no buses going up and down. And when we got out of the car to have a look at it, it was a nice new block but there was a lady looking from the top flat, and it was a tiny little window and it was a little grey head looking out like that, and it gave me the horrors, it looked like a prison. So I said 'no'.

After looking at a few more possibilities that 'didn't look very nice', she came to look at the present scheme and was initially put off by the location, deciding 'no I am never going in sheltered housing'. However, she was persuaded to meet the warden of the scheme where she now lives, who suggested that as she was 'a big lady' with two cats, she might be able to move into a double room with garden space – 'which seemed like a gift, well the council had never done anything like that, you had got to take it or leave it attitude'.

After about a year a suitable flat became available:

I have been here exactly three and a half months. So when [warden] told me about this, she said 'you can have an independent life, I haven't got the time to look after 36 people, so you have all got to be ... it is not a care home, and we don't bother you'. When I moved in I said 'can I do this and do that?' and she said 'you can do what you want' as long as I don't annoy anyone.

Here we see Hermoine scanning the possibilities for improving her situation and, crucially, avoiding the possibility of an 'old people's home'. Clearly not attracted to sheltered housing, she was practically coaxed into it by reassurances about the type of flat she would have, the autonomy she would be able to exercise there and notably the greater spatial flexibility. The key attributes of sheltered housing, on which most people base their decision to move in, are the quality/suitableness of the accommodation; security; and companionship. Yet some of the reservations that been voiced about sheltered housing have included the amount of available space, living just with other older people and the inward-looking social life of such schemes (Percival, 2000). None of our respondents had particular problems with the size of their sheltered flats. Several of them had moved from other small flats and the others had made a conscious trade-off of space for security. Our respondents tended to talk more about the social arrangements in sheltered housing and here respondents from Bedford and Haringey touch on issues of 'cliquishness' and the need for residents to take some initiative in forming social connections:

And ... it is so quiet here, sometimes too quiet. But I have got plenty to do, I have got an elderly man living next door, he has been here a while. He is 82 and he goes and gets a newspaper for me, trots up the road and back, and sometimes we share a jam doughnut and things like that. He is the next flat along. There is only three of us along this corridor. ... It was built for the Irish, and most people are Irish, Irish Roman Catholics, and they stay together. So ... I have managed to get friendly with one or two of them, one lady in particular, a sweet lady. But the others seem to be rather distant. And then there are some that have been here a long time here, not Irish Roman Catholic, Londoners, so they have formed a group. (Hermoine)

We have a common room and that was where my son and daughter came with me when we first looked at the flat and our warden laid on cups of tea and coffee, and generally made us feel very welcome indeed. And I discovered that it wasn't used at all soon after I came, and I thought that was a great pity because generally people living in sheltered housing can be very lonely. And so I was one male with all the ladies at one time, we have rectified that by two more males in [laughs] nothing against the female sex. But I asked the warden, who was very co-operative, whether I could use the common room ... So every Monday morning we use the common room for either table games from 10.30 am–12 pm, and the same for the fellowship group. (Bob)

Hermoine, quoted first, lives in a large scheme with more than 50 flats; Bob in a block of 11. Commenting on how the residents got on together, Bob said, 'Very well. Extremely good warden, which is the key to the whole business. She is one of the best. And we are a small unit, only 11 of us I think in total. So we are a "family".'

In contrast, another of the respondents living in a large sheltered housing scheme felt that its size militated against the formation of real friendships. In this case her sense of disassociation from other people in the scheme was compounded by her disability-standard flat, with direct access to the outside:

I am very happy with my flat, it is a nice flat, but I would pick it up and put it in a smaller building. I would be happier with about 10 people rather than 60 odd flats where you never really make friends, you make lots and lots of acquaintances but to get close to anybody, you don't. Well, I don't perhaps because our ... flat I am in is in a kind of outside block bit, and we have front doors that lead straight outside, and in the other flats in the rest of the building they are leading into a corridor with other flats around you, and you talk to people you know. But in these flats all of them are married couples, except me. And although I know my neighbours I am not close with my neighbours, and I think that is a shame. You know, I would like to have real friends, and they are not real friends, real friends you can just go and talk about anything you know. I am sure they would be there if I was in trouble or anything like that, but it is not the same. Much more difficult to make friends in a big building with people, I think. (Brenda)

Thus the respondents living in sheltered housing identified specific material and organizational factors that they thought affected the likelihood of a thriving community within schemes: the number and disposition of flats; communal facilities; the role of the warden; some commonalities of interest between residents; and the ability of residents to be proactive. While the outsider's perspective may be that residents lead lives of forced introspection or are otherwise inwardly oriented, the expectation from within sheltered housing is that it will facilitate an associative life that residents can opt into and out of and that will provide opportunities for neighbourliness and indeed friendship if that is what people are looking for.

Conclusion

While most older people will succeed in their intention to remain living in their own home and community, using whatever strategies they can to maintain a comfortable enough lifestyle, many nevertheless devise these strategies against a background awareness of alternative, specialized environments for the frail elderly. We have called this 'option recognition'. Popular views of these settings may be stereo-typical, but they are also based on observations of the circumstances of friends, relatives and neighbours; some of the quotations from our respondents in this chapter show this. Their actions were frequently directed at avoiding this stage as well as at maintaining the kind of life they have achieved. While most respondents acknowledge, for the most part, both the amenity and caring benefits of modern residential care homes, these are outweighed by the obvious contrasts between the perceived life of the care home resident and that of people living in the mainstream. These contrasts, as we have seen, centre on observations concerning routines and autonomy. They add up to worries that such environments are not stimulating and that those who inhabit them become under-stimulated and somewhat disengaged.

The data from the small group of informants in residential environments in this study indeed show that the routines of life become less elaborate; choice in companionship becomes compromised; the resident's view of the world outside eventually becomes misty as the internal world becomes amplified. This is a finding that has been repeatedly discussed in the research on residential care settings. The high level of external (to the resident) influence on the design of the residential environment is mirrored by the design of routines into which the resident must fit. While it is true that adapting to other people's routines, such as those of other family members and domiciliary care workers, can seriously restrict the autonomous routine making of people receiving care at home, this is seen, certainly by our respondents, to be more of a problem in the institutional setting.

Current policy is to enable older people to stay at home – i.e. in the mainstream – for as long as possible, but as we have see throughout this book so far the specific attributes of the environment may work for or against older people who wish to take this course. Environmental press will push people towards *option recognition* and many older people will be able to take action but for those who are not able, the press of environment will ultimately require compensatory action, perhaps by carers. But most older people want to optimize their mastery over environment and constantly, if subtly, evaluate their circumstances and, when it appears right to do so, consider the next best step. As part of this process people look for information – formal and informal – to supplement their existing knowledge from their own experiences as well as from stereotypical understandings of what it means to live in specialized environments or to live on at home.

Note

1 See *Care Homes for Older People* (2003), 3rd edn. ISBN 011 3225 79 2, London: The Stationery Office; Proposed Amended Environmental Standards, Care Homes for Older People and Young Adults, 14/03/2003.

7

Living the layered environment

Introduction

Throughout this book we have been looking in different ways at the material in the 'Environment and Identity' study, to focus on time and place, the meaning of the home and its surroundings and how people go about maintaining their identities in 'ordinary' and 'special' housing. We have acknowledged that the analytical division of our data has been necessary to enable us to focus on these themes, but that it inevitably involves the loss of the whole-life context of individuals that is also a significant aspect of the 'Environment and Identity' data. In this chapter, we begin to draw these themes together by looking at how they are presented in specific case studies that indicate the uniqueness of all the 54 respondents.

We present the stories of six people, drawing more extensively on their stories and their own words than we have in previous chapters. Each demonstrates how particular aspects of the environment affect their personal well-being and relate to their continuing identity. They show different aspects of attachment to place and reveal that while the most salient features in the relationship between people and their homes in later life may vary, the importance and subtleties of *option recognition* and re-engagement remains the same. We describe here two men and four women, of whom two live in Haringey, two in Bedford and two in Northamptonshire; the types of home that they live in range from a room in a residential care home to three-bedroomed semi-detached houses (see Figure 7.1).

In demonstrating our study themes within the cases of these six

	Bedford	Northamptonshire	Haringey
Residential care home	x		
Sheltered housing flat			x
Purpose-built bungalow		x	
Semi-detached house		x	x
Semi-detached house with adaptations	x		

Figure 7.1 Case study respondents

individuals, we draw on the whole range of our data, including field notes and structured survey responses (health and finances) as well as on interview transcripts.

Case 1: living in a semi-detached house in a small village

Nerys was aged 73 at interview. Born in Wales, she had moved to Northamptonshire in her early twenties for work and married a widower with a young child who lived in a small village. She had lived there in their family home – a council house that they eventually bought – for 48 years, having two more daughters and suffering the death of twin children in infancy. She had been widowed for less than two years at interview and though having a long history of health problems was active and mobile.

Biographical meaning

> I would not willingly and it would certainly be at the last resort, but I would never willingly leave this house. This house means a great deal; it isn't bricks and mortar to me. It's living, it's real, it's my life, it's my husband's life and my children, it's everything that's near to me and my heart. This furniture came into my house the week before I married and I remember my husband saying, are you sure about this and I said 'yes' this is what I will live from for the rest of my life and I will. I do not like a lot of change, I know what is me. Now I go into people's houses, my

daughter's house is absolutely lovely, all of them, but I wouldn't want to live there, that's not my furniture, that's not my drapes. I'm terribly old fashioned I suppose and also you see we chose them together. It's just everything to me, I mean it's my life, I didn't come here until I was in my mid-twenties, but as I say my husband carried me over the threshold of the door in my wedding dress and I changed here to go on my honeymoon. All my children were born here; I lost my first two children here; my children were married from here; it's a whole life, and my husband died here. So, I could never, never leave it, I shall be in my own little wooden box.

It is clear from listening to Nerys that the specific home and village that she lives in are essential to her well-being and her sense of identity: substitutes for either would not be up to the mark. She had discussed with her children what would happen if she became too ill or frail to continue alone, but the thought of moving was so extreme that she had taken the strategic decision to defer any real consideration of moving until a possible future time of extreme need:

You have got to think about getting older, and I talked to my daughters, and to put it crudely, I do hope that they will take my little wooden box out of here, I do hope. But I do realize you can have strokes, you can be paralyzed and erm . . . I sort of said to them, well then of course I realize I have got to go, but otherwise don't anyone ask me to come and live near them, sort of thing. [Daughter] said to me . . . they have a lovely complex of beautiful flats for elderly people, but you buy them. And she said 'do you know mum, I am not talking about now, but I am talking if you live to be 80 or 90' and I sincerely hope not, I mean not planning to die [laughs]. And she said 'every day I would see you, it is not too far from my home, would you consider it?' and I said 'when it comes to that, we will talk about it dear' but I said 'I don't want your travelling 40 odd miles every day, you have got your own life, you have got your children.' So, she has a pretty busy life. Then I would realize, and I would be sensible enough to do it, I wouldn't want my children to be worn out, I have seen it so many times.

It is notable that, attached as she is to her own home, Nerys was prioritizing her children's needs over her own – and demonstrating the dominant discourse on good parenting that we have discussed in Chapter 2. She also echoed the common theme that health would be the deciding factor in the decision to move – and the tension between children who wish to know that their parents are 'safe' in sheltered housing and the preference of most older people to defer such a move.

In addition to her social links with people in the village, the material environments of the house, garden and village were saturated with biographical meaning for Nerys. Yet inevitably such a close identification with place confers vulnerability as well as security. In spite of the strong emotional support from her home and neighbourhood, Nerys had been finding it very hard to deal with the loss of her husband:

> I am never very late back, I would think the very latest I am back is about 9.45–10.00 pm. But I always have lights on. To be perfectly honest with you it is the one time I really know I am alone, when I come into the house after about 6 pm and that is the time I really feel it .... . So I try very hard to be indoors, and lock up, I always keep my back door locked up, I never used to, but I do now. But not because I am afraid dear, it is the only time I know I am alone. In the day time it is not so bad, but I find the most difficult time for me is from about 4.30–7.00 pm and the one thing I cannot do, is sit around, I have a bath about 6.00 pm and I am in bed by 7.00 pm.

> [*Interviewer:* Is that because you and [husband] would be together?]

> Oh yes. I used to go to bed about 9.30 pm and have a bath and he would get up for 10.00 pm and we would watch the 10 o'clock news, he would be reading the paper and I would do a crossword, and would settle down about 11–11.30 pm. That is how it always was. He went to quite a few meetings but he was always back and we would have a cup of tea and biscuit. And then I would say 'I am off' and he would switch off and come up later. But it is so funny but I cannot sit here at that time and I think to myself it is silly, because I am contented. ... I don't know why. I get through my days. I don't quite know how to explain. It is not the same and it never will be the same, but you have got to get through the days and the nights.

We see here again the salience of routines as temporal anchor points, and the need to re-establish anchors after the disruption of bereavement. As with many of the respondents, Nerys had recognized her own particular times of vulnerability, but for the most part she felt very supported by her environment and believed that this support was the more forthcoming because she had lived for a long time in a village rather than in a town or city.

Village Life

> What's there to be unhappy about walking through this churchyard, an
> awful lot of people I know, friends are here and as you pass you sort of
> think of things that happened. If I lived somewhere ... I suppose it would
> depend on the sort of community spirit that was there, if one lived in
> Kettering for instance and you lived in a row of houses, now do you get
> that same community spirit that you get in a small village, I don't know.
> Perhaps you do, but it would only involve a certain amount of people
> whereas in a small village, it's not just this part of the village but the
> entire village.

Nerys had a very strong sense of community, embracing the past and
the present, and the whole village as one recognizable community with
herself and her late husband as an embedded part of it. In spite of the
heavy blow of the loss of her husband, she was managing a life of
reasonable contentment by remaining very socially active in a neighbourhood that she knew intimately and a home that she loved deeply.
Hers was probably the most clearly articulated example in this study of
a life of quality depending on the continuity of a specific environment.

Case 2: living in a semi-detached house in the city

Hope, aged 89, had lived in the same house in Tottenham, in the
London borough of Haringey, for 62 years. Yet like many London
residents in this generation, her earlier housing history had seen several
moves as a consequence of World War Two – and before that her
father's need to move for work in the coaching trade. She had been
born not too far away in Stoke Newington and had vivid recollections
of her childhood home, in which place and time are inextricably linked
to memories of her younger self:

> I was born in [names] Road, Stoke Newington. I was in number 3. Then
> we moved to number 66 when I was quite a baby. We used to have to go
> along a passage, down a couple of steps to the kitchen and I know I had
> to clean that kitchen every week, so I knew what it was like. We all had
> our little jobs to you, you had to do them or else we didn't get pocket
> money. Pocket money might have been a halfpenny; you were lucky if
> you got a penny.
> And the shops were the other end in Church Street that was, now

Church Street, Stoke Newington, it's called but it was only Church Street. There used to be a little grocer's shop just round the corner and I can remember going in there for a penneth of coconut, I used to love desiccated coconut and I used to get a penneth of coconut there. I can always remember that shop. A few years ago I went down there and everything is different and you know I could say that used to be a so and so; that used to be a greengrocer's just around the corner and you see these different places.

Yes, I can remember the old days more than the new. They mean more to me really.

Hope owns outright her 1930s' three-bedroomed semi-detached house. But when she first moved in, she and her husband rented three ground-floor rooms and a kitchen from the owner. Over time they acquired more of the house and eventually 'struggled and bought it' as sitting tenants. Most of her long life had been lived in this house, where she had raised her own three sons and at various times had other members of her large extended family living with them. She had seen much change in the neighbourhood but had some neighbours she had known for 60 years. She still got out and about with the help of a dial-a-ride service and trips organized by a local social club of which she was a longtime member. The club meets several times a week, although over the years group numbers have dwindled:

Well, you miss people and you think to yourself, well if so and so was there we'd stand and talk ... you don't talk to people now like you used to.

We have the dial-a-ride for the shopping and if we go to the doctors or anything like that they are very good and we have the council people to pick us up Tuesday and Thursday but they don't bring us back, we have dial-a-ride.

Well, I think it works out very well because I don't think I could get up if it wasn't for the dial-a-ride. Because they are very good in helping you and that.

Getting out and staying connected to people was clearly very important to Hope; but given her history in this particular house as the hub of a large family and more recently as its sole occupier, we wanted to probe the nature of her attachment to the house, neighbourhood and community.

Place or people?

I don't think I would be happy to move. That is why the boys don't encourage me to, they say: 'If the time comes mum, well we are all for it, but until then no we won't move you.'

[*Interviewer*: And living here makes you feel ... secure?]

Well, I feel at home.

[*Interviewer*: Can you explain what being at home is made up of?]

Well, I feel I belong here.

[*Interviewer*: Yes.]

I mean where it is as well, at times I feel a bit down, I feel my husband is here, yes. I can always feel the presence of him here.

[*Interviewer*: I mean, say your longstanding neighbour now were to move would that ...?]

It wouldn't worry me. No, because I have never been one for going and visiting. I used to go in and out for her, because she hasn't been out much for years.

[*Interviewer*: So it would be true to say, would it, that you don't depend on these people to be yourself?]

No. No, I don't.

[*Interviewer*: But that might not be true of your family? Your family, you do depend on.]

My family I always feel I can send for them anytime and they will come to me. Yes, I never ... I can always say that they would always see me right.

[*Interviewer*: And your family, and you have got a big family ... in a sense I know they are different to the house, but are they as important as the house in making who you are?]

No. No, the family itself has more play.

[*Interviewer*: The people?]

Yes.

[*Interviewer*: Yes, and then would you say the house comes after?]

After. Oh yes, my boys come first, and their family.

[*Interviewer*: And it is those people who make you who are really.]

Oh yes, every time.

Hope clearly saw the people in her life as more important to her sense of who she was than the place where she lived and in this she was not different from most of our respondents who, in essence, felt the same way. Yet people must live in specific places and as we have seen throughout this book that the physical, social and psychological components of particular places for particular people have a strong effect on whether and how they can maintain both a strong sense of self and satisfactory social relationships. In Hope's case, these environmental supports extend from the dial-a-ride service and the continuity of location-based amenities – important given the changing nature of the community, to the memories associated with her house and the security that ownership of it afforded her.

Case 3: living in a semi-detached house with adaptations, in a large town

Born in Luton 84 years ago, Bertie had lived in Bedford for the last 50 years and was recently widowed. In the early 1990s his wife had suffered a number of strokes that left her disabled. As a retired architect, Bertie decided to use his own design skills to create an environment within their home that would better suit their needs and allow his wife to be cared for at home. These adaptations took place over a period of time and included structural alterations to the house and gardens; experiments with different kinds of off-the-shelf aids and devices; and small tailor-made adjustments to meet specific needs. In talking about this work and about his life before and after the death of his wife, Bertie reveals the interplay between his principal roles in life at this time – husband, friend, carer and professional. Having both the financial ability and knowledge necessary to take this path, Bertie focused on the adaptation of the given environment rather than on other kinds of option such as moving house or looking for residential care.

Adaptation of the physical environment

The first time that his wife was ill, Bertie decided to create an extension and a downstairs toilet so that she could live in the more sociable space of the ground floor. He approached the local social services department for help:

> I had a letter which said that if by any chance we were lucky enough to get a grant I would be expected to pay between £6–7000. Well, I was horrified, so I called the whole thing to a halt and said 'fair enough'. So I went it alone and so I put a shower in myself, I had a lavatory basin put in, took a cupboard out and had the boiler put in the kitchen .... But, she was interested in her clothes and so of course when she wanted to get dressed in the morning, what did I have to do? Go upstairs and I would bring the wrong one down and she said what she wanted and I wouldn't have a clue [laughs] so I trundled up and downstairs and the first thing we did was bring down the wardrobe and stuck it here behind me here. She got all her clothes down here.
>
> One of the things that I don't think is always appreciated is how important access and doors are. You came in this morning through the front wall where the first thing I did was widen it by three feet because if you've got the car in the drive you couldn't push a wheelchair right by it.
>
> I got to the position in the end where the only way to get her out of here [front room] in a chair was to go out through here, through that porch where there was considerable congestion, down a ramp into the garden into a door at the back of the garage, back through the garage right around the front wall ... it was a major issue.
>
> You know going to church on a Sunday morning and then she would want to go to the toilet at the last minute and then people are looking at you when you are getting late and it takes you ages to do this sort of operation, going out was a major issue. So I decided we can't go on like this – we'd get jammed with the chair in that back door couldn't get her in or out and I thought I'd have to change the drive. A pattern was created at the front to get her in. I'd widen the drive, then the question of height came into it. She couldn't negotiate the steps, so I did a ramp myself which went up one side so that you could get a wheelchair up and I adjusted the steps a bit so that you could also walk in and there was a rise between so that she had the option. She wasn't embarrassed by the fact that everything pointed to the fact that her being incapacitated.
>
> You can see yourself if you're with a person and perhaps that's where I had the advantage on the OT, I was with her all the while so I could see whether a handle was needed and one of the vital ones is at the top of the

stairs on the newel post as you get off the stair lift, at the top of the stairs, you have a handle to grasp . . . .

Upstairs we've got a toilet and the very same situation arose, I put handles both sides, but then you've got a 2′6″ door swing in and you sterilize 2′6″ of the floor space and so I put bi-fold doors up there and I did the same in the bathroom because there we wanted additional room. You see it wasn't only the patient, we wanted a carer alongside her and there wasn't room or if there was room the door swing was in the way, so I put bi-fold doors in there.

I would say that the authorities have been very helpful, but I do believe that a lot of things . . . if you do have the inclination to be a do it yourself, you can do it yourself and I have done a lot, I shouldn't say it really, but I have. I mean, even raising the height of a thing, I mean I have got a milk bottle carrier outside the back door, it is a nonsense really it has been up years, but instead of having to bend down to pick my milk up I put my hand out and it is at the right level.

Adaptation to living alone

As Bertie acknowledged, he was still in the process of adjusting to life after the death of his wife and in addition to personal bereavement he was dealing with a drastic change in the focus of his daily activities and in his routines. This brought new freedoms to take his own time, arrange things to suit his own needs and become more engaged in old interests: for example, he had recently replaced his piano after 75 years – with no regrets. Both time and space had expanded for Bertie and he was working out ways to deal with them:

Yes, I mean I can get up whatever time I like. One of my worries is that if my curtains aren't drawn certain neighbours of mine are wondering what is happening [laughs] and they will come and diplomatically tap the front window or door. I am grateful for that. ... In fact, I have an arrangement whereby as a result of difficulties caused my neighbour this way, I would draw the side curtain so that they would know I was on the move [laughs]. So if I decide I don't want to get up at the moment that means it is sometimes 10 am before I start moving.

One thing people have said to me 'are you going to move?' and I won't move until we have got buses on the doorstep [in an alternative location] really, the church is near, people you know are here, I have got a son ... not far away, they were here last night with two of his girls. I don't know, some things in life you don't know until you face them do you?

We go through life where we haven't got enough room, extensions here, there, and everywhere, and then you get to a point in life where you want to shrink everything really, although you can never have too much space. It is like a greenhouse, it is never big enough .... I don't go in the other two bedrooms much, but I use everything else. And because this business of in here you ... I can pull this across but you can never achieve the privacy you might need if you wanted it, but for comfort and warmth you can pull the screen across. But no, I live ... and, in fact, I deliberately don't stay in one room .... I think that would be such a big mistake. Like sitting in my posh chair, they said to me last night 'why aren't you sitting in your chair?' and I said 'well I don't sit in that all the while' [laughs]. It is a lovely thing when you press a button and your feet start to come up, at the end of the day.

We see in this last quotation an articulation of a need we have described elsewhere (Kellaher et al, 2004), for older people to have the capacity to move from and to their emotional and functional 'anchor' point in order to maintain mastery over and interest in their environment. At different levels, Bertie knew this was important – whether getting out and about in his car, using different parts of the house, or just varying where he chose to sit, he was maintaining routines without getting into a rut. In talking about what matters in his environment, he also brings up some of the issues about internal space, transport and neighbouring that we have discussed at various points in this book. In this final quote from Bertie, he talks about his relationship with the natural world: the park outside the house and his own garden and the pet birds he keeps in it. It gives an indication of the importance to him of remaining connected with the environment and with other people – living alone and with increasing health problems, he has a strong sense of the inadvisability of becoming focused too much on himself.

I get so much pleasure, look at the trees now ... I take photographs when the snow is on the ground, you see the children on their trays or egg boxes, whatever. And you see people ... you don't see a lot of people up here, that is one thing. ... But I am so puzzled that some people don't seem to be aware of what is around them, because as far as I am concerned the garden, I try to put shrubs in that have got winter value, flowers on. And they are astonishing, I only planted those five weeks ago and look at them now, something has gone wrong! I get a lot of pleasure of messing around. [late wife] said she wanted some budgerigars two or three years ago, and I said 'are you serious?' and she knew as a boy I used to keep them, and so she said she did, and so I thought I would make an aviary, and so I built an aviary and having built it I realized it was fundamentally wrong so I had to virtually rebuild it, and we had about a dozen birds up there, which you can see from here. But, I sometimes wonder whether we should have them there, because once a month I have to feed them. I am getting lazy aren't I? I will tell you one thing that is worrying, and I said it only recently, one of the things with living on your own, it can make you very selfish .... I am certain that is the case. I have seen it in other people, I suppose it is easy to do that than see it in yourself. But instead of having to think about the result of this or that, you only think about yourself, and that can be so selfish.

Case 4: living in a purpose-built bungalow in a small town

Nancy was aged 77 at interview. Asked where she felt she belonged, she said: 'I am Burtoner folk now ... I think I have been here long enough now.' Born in Northampton, Nancy had experienced hostel life in the World War Two land army before she married and moved in the early 1950s to the smaller town of Burton Latimer and a new three-bedroomed council house, one of the first to be built locally after the war. At the end of the 1980s, she moved with her husband to her present accommodation: a purpose-built retirement bungalow, also rented from the council. This has two bedrooms and a bathroom plus (for the first time in their marriage) central heating and all doors are wide enough for a wheelchair. However, her husband had died within 18 months of moving to the bungalow and she had now been widowed for about 12 years. Nancy suffers from several long-term limiting conditions including osteoporosis and had recently broken a femur, limiting her mobility.

Neighbourhood change

> When I first came it was only a little tiny place – we'd got our own police station, the sergeant and three policemen; we'd got our own electric office, gas office everything and there were four or five shoe factories, about three clothing factories; two engineering places ... I mean there was never any need for anybody to go out of town to work. People used

to come into Burton to work, but now there's nothing, there's no shoe factories; no clothing factories. You've still got the Weetabix factory but there's not a lot of what used to be. Most people go out of the town to work, there are little pockets of employment, little tiny factories that have grown up but nothing to speak of. Of course, we've got no police station now, you never see policemen the same as everybody else you know.

Option recognition

Nancy had been consciously considering her housing options since around the time that she and her husband retired. When a new development of houses was built at the far end of the village, they were aware that it included rented bungalows for older people and they applied to move into one. They were offered a property on a hillside where the front entrance was partly obscured by a wall:

> When I first saw it behind the wall, I said 'Oh if it's behind that wall I'm not going behind there, I'm not going to be shut behind there ...' But when we walked in and saw how nice and light and that we saw this room looking onto the garden – which then was a tip like sort of thing, but I thought 'oh yes that will do, we'll come here' and of course, we were only here just over a year when my husband died unfortunately so ...
>
> Well, I mean ... at the moment I am alright as I am. I did think about moving because I wanted a walk-in shower, because I cannot get .... I mean before my husband died I couldn't get in the bath ... well, I could but you couldn't get out. But then when he died I thought I couldn't have a bath, so my son fixed a shower up over the bath. But now since I have done this, and my back again, I can't get in to have a bath. And I have put in to the council to see whether I could have a walk-in shower, but oh no that was it, I am not disabled enough. They wouldn't even consider it .... I don't know how you are supposed to be before you get one of them, crawling on your hands and knees I think, but that is besides the point ...

When asked about the possibility of moving into sheltered housing:

> No, not now. I did think about it, had a chance to have a flat in [sheltered housing scheme] and that is ... there's not a warden actually lives there but you've got the emergency bells you know if you wanted any help or anything but er I had the chance of one, I went, my friend lives in one, and the one she's in is on the opposite side of the building and you look all over the fields and it's lovely, you know it's really nice and bright and sunny. But this one I went to see that I got the chance of it was on

the other side of the building just looking at the walls of the other flats and it was dark and dreary and as soon as I walked in I thought oh no that's not for me. I'd have to let me daughter have the dog 'cos you know you're not allowed animals there . . . . My home means everything, mine, I mean it's well it's not mine, it's the council bungalow but you know . . . I really am fond of my little bungalow and my dog . . .

I know a heck of a lot of people. But . . . I don't know, I love my big patio windows and I can see the weather and see my garden, and you know down there you have got smaller windows and I think I would get a bit claustrophobic if I went down there. Although it is right in the middle of Burton, so I know this isn't far but it is far enough when you are in pain, you know. I don't know . . . I will weigh it up. I might consider it actually if I hadn't got the dog, but I don't think I want to part with her, bless her.

[*Interviewer*: So might that make the difference, if the dog went would that tip the balance the other way?]

I think it would yes. Yes, I think it might actually. Because as I say I know everybody down there so it is no problem, and it is right on the doorstep for my clubs and social activities as they are [laughs].

This discussion clearly shows the processes that can be involved in decisions about whether, when and where to move. It is rarely a simple matter and older people in this position – settled and attached to their home, but aware of encroaching problems – must make fine judgements as they constantly scan their options. Nancy considered change and decided against it . . . for now. But she knows that at some future point the benefits of moving may come to outweigh the losses. Should the right flat become available – one that allows her to live the life of quality that she has so far maintained – the fact that the sheltered housing scheme would bring her closer to the centre of her small town, and to her friends, is a very important consideration.

Support

In the meantime, Nancy manages her disability with the help of friends and support services that make it possible for her to continue living in her present home and maintain it to acceptable standards. They also make it possible for her to get out of the house for shopping and to maintain a social and cultural life in the town:

I love my garden it's just big enough for me, until I got osteoporosis and then I fractured my femur it was ... I could do it myself ... but I can't get down to do it now and me neighbour helps, he has to come and do it now, it's very kind of him, so that gets done. I ... I've started putting things in pots and I can have a potter round myself ...

I can walk for about a quarter of an hour I should think and then I have to have a little sit but you know coming back is the worst, up the hill you know. Walking up that hill from the Old Vic it starts you know – the pub at the bottom there ... it's a bit of a drag especially if you've got shopping but I don't carry a lot of shopping because either my neighbour fetches things for me if I need anything heavy or my relatives take me shopping you know, so I manage.

So we have a local taxi down and he pick us up about an hour later. On Thursdays we go down usually, and pay our rent, pick our pension up, have a little waddle round Gateway, you know, do a bit of shopping, and go and have a cup of coffee in Crumbs, and he comes and picks us up there and brings us home again [laughs]. Then we go to our clubs, on Monday it is the Monday Club, Fridays we've got Derby and Joan. One Monday a month in the evening we go to the British Legion, and we usually have taxis then, but he don't charge much.

I used to go every Tuesday morning to [church]. That is 9–10 am it is a communion, but I am afraid I haven't been lately because of kneeling down and getting up [laughs] you know. You sit down, but I know it isn't the same, it might seem silly, but it don't seem the same ...

I do have a little lass on Fridays, she comes and hoovers all through for me, that's about the only thing really that I can't manage you know because I can't push the hoover and walk on a stick at the same time ... and sort of climbing up to change a light bulb or anything simple like that you know I can't do that but either my neighbour or my son-in-law when he comes over does things for me. Oh I've got plenty of help. I've got some good friends and neighbours – not too bad ...

Here we see that the support that Nancy is able to martial enables her to maintain autonomy and the routines that she has worked out, as we have described in Chapter 5, fundamentally support her sense of control over her own life. Only in the case of the church ritual do we get a hint of defeat where she has drawn back from an accustomed routine because of her disability.

Case 5: living in sheltered housing

Harjit, aged 66 at interview, had been born in India and brought up in Bombay, moving as a young man to Scotland as a student, and subsequently living in various parts of the UK (including parts of the Midlands) before settling in London. Twice divorced, Harjit was currently living alone in a large local authority sheltered housing scheme in Haringey. Although Indian by origin, he had lived in Britain for almost all his adult life and negotiated his identity between two cultures. His medical history included two serious accidents that had left him with mobility and health problems which continued to affect his options.

Health

> I got in touch with the local authority and social services when I had the second accident. My thigh bone was broken and when I was in hospital and when I came out and all that I contacted them and again I was in a wheelchair and couldn't walk. This was a building that was newly built and I was accepted ... I had a look at it yes, and I liked it especially the arrangement where, if I am in trouble I can pull a cord and call some assistance which is very good, and it's a fairly secure place.

At the time of his accident, Harjit had been living in a place that he already found difficult because of stairs and his clear priority had been to secure accommodation that would allow him to remain independent in spite of his mobility and health problems. He had chosen his present home particularly for its offer of security and very importantly because it was located within reach of healthcare. Subsequently, the location of the flat, relative to specific healthcare, became essential:

> I go to Bart's Hospital for my heart, Royal London Hospital for my kidneys, Middlesex for my eyes and my diabetes, also my GP is in Tottenham.

Belonging

Harjit had ambiguous feelings about the degree to which he belonged in the UK and in India. He dealt with this ambiguity by surrounding himself with links to Indian culture, while acknowledging that his work and social lives and his housing history had resulted in effective attachments in the culture where he had lived longest:

In many ways mentally and in my thinking processes I am more like British but culturally I am Indian, so I am in a sort of limbo, in between. So I could say that I belong to both of them or none of them, completely. So it's just one of those states you've got to make the best of the situation and adapt yourself.

... to be truthful, many people like us here who after being here for such a long time, if you go to India we are out of place there because India has evolved and developed in a different direction and a different way to the way we have done here. In other words we have got British values, it is not only the language but other things as well about law, standards and other things. And we are out of place there. We don't belong there, you see. And that is why ... and sometimes at odd times we feel we don't belong here, so we are in limbo sort of thing, you get that feeling. But most of the time I feel this is my home ... we take part in politics, we back a football team, we do anything that any British citizen would do, which when you go to India we are foreigners. And it stands out a mile.

Recently, quite a few years now, there have been Indian channels in Britain, television channels and radios and I've got two Indian channels on my television which are directly from India so I get the news and entertainment and everything – what they get, I get and so it's not too bad – it's like being in India when you are watching that ...

These quotes show how Harjit had, over many years, steered a course between two cultures to arrive at a position of relative comfort. Even if he did not always feel that he completely belonged where he lived, he knew that moving would probably not bring benefits. His best option was to use other means to integrate aspects of his personality that were not adequately expressed in the given environment. He therefore brought aspects of Indian culture into his home including TV channels, objects and a Hindu shrine (conveniently tucked inside a wardrobe) and, in addition, he had developed a network of friends for mutual support.

Social support

Well, I have got good friends, over the years I've helped people who are less fortunate than I am and they help me in return by sometimes coming with me for shopping or doing my shopping or doing some things that I can't do myself like lifting and putting rubbish out or anything like that all sorts of things heavy. So they do that in return and I do these things [paperwork] for them. So it's working out very nicely at the moment.

I keep to myself [within the sheltered housing scheme] more or less for two reasons; they're mostly women, and the second thing is mostly they are not academic or educated or anything like that, and the third thing is their interests and everything are different. ... I used to go down and associate with them, but lately since the luncheon club has closed down I have kept to myself more or less. But ... I have got my other friends outside who help me with disposing of my newspapers for recycling, getting my shopping in, or any other heavy work I want to do, and so many other things you know. I have known them for ages. ... My two or three friends they phone me nearly every day to make sure I am alright. And I go to their houses as well. And these people come to my house to visit me. And any time I want anything they are quite happy to help out.

Although Harjit had been a house owner at an earlier period of his life, his housing history as a whole had been marked by disruptive relocations related to migration, divorce and disabling accidents. His present rented flat suited his needs well in most respects. He relied on his motability car to be mobile beyond the sheltered housing complex and had found that when he could not use it (because of an icy pathway) he was confined to the building. He did not feel strongly embedded in the social life of the complex but continued to maintain his social life beyond it. Harjit recognized that this environment, while not perhaps what he would have envisaged for himself, enabled him to manage his health needs, reflect the Indian and British aspects of his identity and continue to live a life which satisfied him on his own terms.

Case 6: living in a residential care home for older people

Bronwyn, aged 93 at interview, had been born in Sheffield, the second of four children of whom she was now the only survivor. She had lived in Bedfordshire since her marriage as a young woman. Before that, she was in domestic service as a housemaid in rural Yorkshire:

There was not much else to do in those villages. When I was married we came back and got a house in Luton. I worked at the hospital in ... the Luton & Dunstable. I was in the sewing room, sewing names on the coats and things like that .... It was a rented house. I haven't had a house in Bedford. I had a house in Luton and when my husband died my daughter wanted me to come and live with her, and I came to live with her.

For a while (she is not sure how long), Bronwyn lived in her daughter's house, with her own bedroom: 'It was with the family, it was just a bed and I could go up to it when I wanted to, which wasn't very often. And I came to live here because my daughter's husband was taken ill. ... And it was an option, I mean it was a case of it had to be. And er ... I have no regrets.'

At the time of interview, Bronwyn had been living in this residential care home in Bedford for about 12 years. She likes to spend most of her days in company, usually just going back to her room at bedtime. Bronwyn is considered to be frail and she needs help with getting dressed and undressed and getting up and going to bed. Yet she clearly takes an optimistic view of her health and mobility. She considers her health to be

[Q]uite good really. I have had operations for different things but ... I got over them. I am not in a wheelchair all the time, I have wheels that I walk about with. But I couldn't do without them at all. I mean, I go in the wheelchair and they take me to the park and that. [Her hearing is] not as good as it might be, sometimes you know if there are too many people talking I don't catch what they are saying you know, but other than that it is ok [she has drops in her eyes twice a day], but apart from that, with glasses I am alright.

Routines

Over time, Bronwyn's range of activities has become increasingly restricted. She relies on staff to help her to move around the home. There is a garden but she tends to sit in it only in the summer. She reads newspapers and books and watches television, but doesn't listen to the radio. On Wednesdays she takes part in the weekly bingo session, but: 'That is about all really. I read. You can have your visitors when you want, they come whenever.' Her daughter comes to visit almost every day, and her son comes once a week. She used to spend every weekend at her son's house, but: 'I come back here to sleep now because it is difficult to get upstairs. I don't stay weekends now because of ... it is not convenient.' Perhaps she is hinting delicately here at problems of access to a toilet as well as a bedroom. She does occasionally get out of the home, for example if taken shopping: 'My daughter would take me, probably, to Milton Keynes. Because Bedford is no good with a wheelchair. There is too many ups and downs .... Oh yes, I enjoy going around the shops, having a look at what is going on [laughs].'

Bronwyn's zest for interesting things to see and for people to talk to is evident from this remark and from her liking of different kinds of food and her habit of spending her time, until quite late (10 pm) at night, in company. This taste for being 'where the action is' is juxtaposed with the ingrained routine of life in the residential care home. For example Bronwyn usually sits in the same lounge, in the same chair:

[*Interviewer*: Why would you use that lounge?]

Because I have got a chair there, that usually ... sometimes there is someone in it, but ... you sit in another chair and wait for it, but you usually keep to your own chairs.

Belongings

When Bronwyn moved to the residential care home, she was able to bring a small selection of her furniture. For some time the rest of her belongings stayed in her old room in her daughter's house, and in this sense she still 'had' the room and her possessions. However, her daughter, now retired, was about to move herself into a bungalow. Bronwyn's furniture and possessions were therefore being distributed to the grandchildren or otherwise disposed of. Her daughter needed more manageable accommodation for her own old age and here we see again that such accommodation eliminates the space for her to keep her mother's things together. However, Bronwyn is not unhappy about this because she had lived without her possessions for such a long time that she had grown less attached to them. She does have family photos and some small ornaments and these were arranged neatly in the room. Bronwyn has to rely on other people to take care of her body, her financial affairs (she has no idea how much it costs to stay here), her routines and her clothes; but these small objects are manageable and within reach, so that she can continue to care for a small but symbolically significant portion of her material world.

Living in a residential care home

The bedroom is just about large enough for the bedroom furniture and a sink and when Bronwyn comes into the room in a wheelchair, there is no circulation space at all. The room is quiet, warm and cosy and has a nice view of the garden. Is there anything about the room she would like to change? 'Not really, I don't think. I can't move about too much anyway to ... you know, I am quite happy to get in my room, get into my bed. I mean, the staff are nice, and ... I get on with most of them, I don't think there is any problems.' Bronwyn says that she is never lonely in the home and she feels that she can be herself. Asked what the best thing is about living there, she replies:

> About living here? ... Well I don't have to think for myself, organizing and everything, it is all done for me. And what they don't do, my daughter does.

> [*Interviewer*: Do you find that quite restful now?]

> Oh yes, yes, yes. I couldn't be bothered to do anymore. Because you know how old I am?

Bronwyn considers herself to be a cheerful person, but not one that feels herself to be inferior to others. She likes to make her own mind up and can get angry if she feels she is not being treated properly. Yet she is happy now to 'take things as they come' and delegate bothersome decisions to other people. In this, Bronwyn is conserving her energy for the things that interest her as her bodily capabilities gradually decline. Fully accepting of her situation, Bronwyn finds that she is in the right place for this stage of her life where she has disengaged from the inessential – allowing others to do the caring about her quality of life – so that she can retain her ability to engage with those things that continue to generate a life of some quality for her.

Conclusion

These six cases give a flavour of the kinds of conversation we had with all the respondents in the 'Environment and Identity' study, but even here we cannot present anything like the whole story of these six people's complex relationships with their home environments. The headings under which we have discussed particular aspects of the respondents' interviews are far from exhaustive and for all the respondents there are many strands of thought weaving in and out of their accounts of past and present homes and the things that are important to them. Our analysis of the everyday lives of older people living in a variety of settings and locations has taken us away from the more structured measurement and assessment of the concept of quality of life to a far more holistic understanding of the elements that go to make a 'life of quality'. In the final chapter of this book we draw together some of these themes and consider the implications of our analysis for our understanding of theory on environment in later life.

8

Environmental biography: tracing the self

The six older people whose lives we touch on in Chapter 7 begin to tell us something of the different layers of environment in which any life is embedded. By using the 'facets of life wheel', conversations with our informants were directed to specific issues and yet the complexity of people's stories led us to consider concerns that reflect aspects of material, social and psychological environment, at levels that are both micro and macro, and often intertwined.

We are conscious that by encouraging an open definition of environment the understanding of place can take very different paths. In our study, some people were living in age-segregated housing with different levels of formal care, while the majority maintained their lives in mainstream housing. Their experiences highlight different issues. In our ageing population different generations are facing what we have called 'option recognition', with implications for how they are able to engage with place. In the previous chapter, the comments of Bronwyn, in her nineties, on leaving her daughter's home for a residential care home show how a person may welcome others having taken on the responsibility for organizing life's routines allowing them to disengage as they wish. In contrast, the impact of globalization is reflected in Harjit's feelings of 'living in limbo' while finding ways of aligning two cultures within his current lifestyle; showing how he can make supported living meet his needs. Nancy, living in a purpose-built bungalow, makes the first tentative moves to consider more supportive accommodation but puts this 'on hold' because the proposed environment does not suit her needs or accommodate her close relationship with her dog. Bertie's *option recognition* extended to his own ability to support his wife during poor health by using his architectural skills. The adaptations he has made also enable him to consider his own environmental needs. Nerys' intense attachment to home and village as an embodiment of her married life and partnership displays both strengths and vulnerability and Hope's maintenance of locational continuity provides the historical context for the people/place interaction that maintains her well-being. Their complex accounts reflect just some of the 54 environmental biographies on which we base our conclusions regarding the relationship between environment and identity.

Reflecting on methodology

It was always our aim to develop a qualitative methodology and while we did not adopt the level of detail in the ethnographic methods of Rowles and Rubinstein, as outlined in Chapter 1, we acknowledge the importance of detail that needs to be drawn from engaging with people for long periods of time and observing their daily life.

During the ESRC's: Growing Older programme time was taken to discuss the concept of 'quality of life' that underpinned all the projects. Researchers considered how this has been assessed and measured within more systematic and quantitative research and what can be learned from more qualitative approaches (Walker and Hagan Hennessy, 2005). As Bowling (2004) has shown, measures said to reflect 'quality of life' are seen to encompass: health status, functional ability, psychological well-being; social networks, life satisfaction and morale. 'Environment' in material and social forms directly or indirectly affects all of these facets, but the psychological interaction between environment and identity, as cumulative, is less easy to assess through the formality of ADL and other psychometric assessments. By adopting an ethnographic approach to the research we have been able to understand how people create, or constantly try to create, a life of quality that meets their expectations. In doing so, we consider our question: *How far can the layered environment be drawn on to reflect the complex self in later life?*

In this sense, we have moved away from earlier work in environmental gerontology, which saw the material environment as becoming more stressful as a person's physical or mental competence declined.

Our understanding of 'what is the person/environment fit?' has to encompass a life history approach.

On reflection we see that we have begun to follow the course discussed by Kaufman (1986, 2000) in her consideration of identity in *The Ageless Self*. She states:

> The construction of a coherent, unified sense of self is an ongoing process. We have seen how old people express an identity through themes which are rooted in personal experience, particular structural factors, and a constellation of value orientations ... The sources of meaning which themes integrate are continually reinterpreted in light of new circumstances. A person selects events from his or her past to structure and restructure his or her identity. Thus, themes continue to evolve from and give form to personal experience – making identity a cumulative process. (Kaufman, 1986 p.104)

How can factors related to environment help to shape such themes? Whilst we, the researchers, chose the domain of environment for examination, through our conversations the respondents set the agenda and the way that they responded tells us something about the validity of our approach to the topic. Initially, we had defined environment in the broadest possible fashion allowing our respondents to operationalize this concept in their own way. In essence, we could not assume that environment, in encapsulating daily living, is just the context in which events happen and within which the self is situated; and while we had expected the 'home' to be a central talking point, we were unsure as to its centrality.

What has emerged in this dataset is a layering of environment that reveals its complexity. We noted in Chapter 1 that Lawton spoke of how environment, if not perceived by older people as stressful, could be 'tuned out' at the level of comfort that was experienced unconsciously or indeed recognized with pleasure. We invited people to speak of this and their commentaries reveal the richness of the everyday. In Chapters 2 to 6, we discussed different aspects of environmental meaning that recognize the diversity of experience. We started by focusing on lifelong experiences seen through housing histories, showing how for some people place is intimately linked to 'significant others' who may have influenced or controlled where and how people have lived. Issues of generation, gender, social class and ethnicity are revealed through these data and we can see the paths of 'migrants', 'movers' and 'locals'. The dialectic of autonomy and security is also played out across these histories as people negotiate location, tenure and types of accommodation creating lifestyle changes that continue into later life and as people contemplate the situation of the end of life. Chapter 3 recognizes the uniqueness of location, discussing people's views on whether they feel that they are in the 'right place' in later life. Living in cities, towns and villages raises questions of people in places, population density and how the older person experiences community living. Many of our respondents report that their experiences of community are in some ways confined by accessibility and limited by time and opportunity. A majority do not go out at night and they are conscious of neighbourhood change that leads many of them to comment on crime and security. For some, this has become a lifestyle that we have called 'integrated segregation' where people are a part of the wider society but their engagement becomes more localized and particularly dependent on access to transport. This is a form of social exclusion that may or may not be a chosen one.

Nearer to home, we consider comments on the natural environment, recognizing the value of flora and fauna in providing solace; and of the value of activity and engagement through surveillance. The garden may offer an opportunity to display expertise and provide a sanctuary for relaxation or participation without pressure. However, the garden may also be felt as an environmental press and a number of respondents commented on how it had become a problem; a potential indicator displayed to all that they were not coping as well as they once had. For a few, a garden or surroundings that were poorly maintained prompted *option recognition* in terms of thinking about relocation. However, very few respondents living in mainstream housing admitted to thinking seriously about moving in old age. Their everyday concerns dwelt on getting through the day in ways that were scheduled, mentally and physically, by routines and plans that enabled them to engage with the material environment of their housing as well as the wider world. The rhythm of life defines the self in interactions with the fragmented spaces of the home. Our respondents knew how and where they wished to spend their time and the pace at which they could engage. They might enjoy interruptions to their routines and unexpected pleasures, but in the main had expectations about visits from and to their families and friends. The issues of time and space are developed further below.

It is through our discussion of living in mainstream housing that we are able to make comparisons with those who have moved into age-segregated accommodation. We have called this chapter 'pacing the self' for we feel that this is what people do. They may think about their futures but defer action. While they are not waiting for a crisis to occur and make that decision for them, they also realize that relocation to 'special' housing will make them 'special' and in the main this is not what they want. However, the rhetoric of 'being a burden' to family members often hangs over people and for some it may also foreshadow end-of-life care. Throughout this discussion we are aware of tensions between issues of security, companionship, autonomy, frailty, dependence, independence. Sometimes personal identity may be affected by stereotypes attached to places such as care homes.

It is not until Chapter 7 that we have given detailed consideration to the environmental biographies of six respondents living in housing that includes mainstream and special accommodation across the three locations. By focusing on a few individuals, we begin to see how a number of factors, recognized in the wider sample, link environment to identity and it is to these factors that we now turn.

Place identity

Can an attachment to, or situation within, a place support or develop a person's identity? In discussing the concept of place identity, Twigger-Ross and Uzzell (1996) explore four factors, following the work of Breakwell (1986, 1992, 1993), that they suggest unpack this topic: distinctiveness; continuity; self-esteem and self-efficacy. We utilize these to address environment and identity in later life. The principle of *distinctiveness* or *uniqueness* has already been noted. Our respondents lived within the city, town, suburbia and villages. It was not a common response but a few said that they saw themselves as Londoners, people of Bedford or a 'Burtoner' (from Burton Latimer, Northamptonshire). For people who know these locations, this type of comment suggests a certain type of lifestyle that is common to all and transcends issues that may relate to age. It can be seen as being grounded and reflects a sense of belonging.

However, in contrast we can also comment on how distinctiveness can be applied to the ways in which people may be associated with particular forms of accommodation seen as 'special' and age segregated, which can occur in any location. In reflecting on Laws' consideration of the spatiality of ageing outlined in Chapter 1, we note that particular locations may be more socially exclusive and consequentially impact on collective stereotypes. The comment: 'I hope I never do, I hope I die before I go into an old people's home' (Naomi) reflects the negative distinctiveness with which older people can associate end of life in care homes (Katz and Peace, 2003). However, as shown in Chapter 6, those resident in care homes in this study varied in their contentment with their situation, from those who knew that they were not 'in the right place' to those who had accepted the 'organized life' as allowing them to focus on self. This suggests the need for further examination of how people are able to remain in what they cognitively and materially construct and reconstruct as the 'right place'.

A second factor in developing place identity is *continuity* through association with place where it continues to remind a person of a past life that maintains and develops the continuity of the self. For long-term residents the housing and the place itself may form constant reminders of their lives. Indeed, as we saw in the case of Nerys, deeply attached to her home and village, maintenance of continuity could well become all embracing. Of course the other side of continuity is change and loss and the discussion of housing histories has highlighted the diversity that exists in continuity of place for these respondents. The experience of relocation across the life course will affect a person's capacity to cope with change. Twigger-Ross and Uzzell refer to Hormuth's (1990) suggestion that 'choosing to move can represent self-concept change with the old place becoming a symbol of the old self and the new place representing an opportunity to develop new identities' (1996, p.207). As noted earlier, control over relocation including the maintenance of key possessions is important for maintaining psychological well-being; a factor that has been identified in relation to older people moving to care homes (Willcocks et al., 1987).

It is also true that people may seek to relocate to places that they feel are congruent with aspects of self in order to maintain some aspect of continuity. There were few examples of such congruent relocations in this study where respondents had recently moved; although in the case of Nancy, it was obvious that she had moved locally within the same village to an environment in which she felt 'at home'. A good example of such continuity can be seen in Kellaher's (2000) study of people living in Methodist care homes where mutuality based on religious faith was apparent. If relocation to places that offer congruence with the self are not possible, people may be able to modify their environment in order to make the environment more fitting for them. Everyday adaptations are common and Bertie, seen in Chapter 7, gives a clear example of how it has been possible for someone to adapt the family housing to suit his wife's needs and maintain continuity of self within place.

The two final characteristics of place identity discussed here are *self-esteem* – whether a specific place makes a person 'feel good about themselves' – and *self-efficacy* – whether the environment is manageable and enables someone to maintain their daily lifestyle. In the main, these two aspects of place identity were acknowledged by respondents living in mainstream housing and also within sheltered housing. Indeed, it was true that for some respondents moving to sheltered housing had led to an improvement in both self-esteem and self-efficacy. Horace, who was interviewed in a care home where he had been sent for rehabilitation following a hospital stay, could not wait to leave. While he recognized that he may no longer be able to maintain his previous lifestyle, he was aware that the care home was affecting both his self-esteem and self-efficacy so that he was looking for a compromise in sheltered housing.

Time and space

The environmental biographies of people living in a variety of mainstream homes show us how daily lives involve activities that display temporal and spatial fragmentation. During the course of any one day people move through their routines, which lead them to engage with different parts of their home, their surroundings, their neighbourhood and beyond. Engagement and integrative actions within these spaces depend on there being 'anchor points' of association over which they maintain control. People may be used to doing something a certain way in a certain place, and the autonomy of everyday lives is achieved through constant engagement and re-engagement with the self, which can intend and execute wishes. Our data are sympathetic to the psychosocial processes linking person to place which Rubinstein (1989) identified since they show how our respondents identify their autonomous selves through establishing their own level of quality in life.

The 'Environment and Identity' study has permitted comparability between people living in diverse accommodation, mainstream and age segregated, which allows for subtle exploration of the differences between settings. It is when a level of environmental mastery begins to fail that a sense of and reaction to environmental press may be observed. In the main, people will attempt to cope with such press through adaptation, reorganization, the introduction of increased support and finding ways to maintain their level of control. It is during these periods that some people may begin to embark on *option recognition*, possibly leading to relocation in supported housing. At this point characteristics of gender, social class and ethnicity may combine with age to influence the real options available within different locations. These characteristics also affect the perceived normalcy of different forms of accommodation. In this study, sheltered housing was the mainstay of older people's public housing in Haringey and consequently *option recognition* in this location could include sheltered housing as a not unusual choice. Indeed, for many Haringey residents who had been longstanding occupants of social housing, such a move could sometimes enhance self-esteem and self-efficacy.

While the material environment may change, spatial and temporal fragmentation and the following of routines continue, along with the impulse to bring these components together. Where this was the case, people were able to continue leading relatively autonomous lives within an environment that provided a level of security that could enhance well-being. The importance of maintaining a place of comfort from which to direct life seems to be crucial to the maintenance of identity.

In this study, it was not until older people, often those of advanced age, come to live in care homes that they experienced an environment lacking both the spatial and temporal variation that generates the fragmentations that characterize daily life in the mainstream. While it is true that the experience of older people currently living in care homes may involve more person-centred care and less institutional practices, these remain organized environments where the working lives of staff are paced in such a way as to take over agency and wrest power from residents. Older people find it hard to remain autonomous and therefore we argue to engage with the self in situations where routine and space are integrated by others and other forces outside their control. Elsewhere we have argued for person-centred care that facilitates ways of enabling older people to remain as autonomous as possible within care settings (Peace et al., 1997). While this should remain a goal where people wish for this minimal level of engagement, we also recognize that at the end of life temporal and spatial needs may be overshadowed by more essential needs of the self. We believe that this type of in-depth research should also be applied to other situations in which older people may find themselves living, from the co-housing scheme to the retirement community (Brenton, 2001; Phillips et al., 2001), where the opportunity for different lifestyles has a bearing on the creation of fragmented spaces and times and the consequent capacity for activity.

Environment and identity in later life

At the beginning of this book we asked the question: 'Does where you are affect who you are?' Through in-depth interviews with people who saw themselves as 'older' in their 60s, 70s, 80s and 90s, we have been able to learn about how they perceive the environments in which they live and whether they feel that it impacts on how they see themselves. The accounts upon which we have drawn in this study indicate the many layers that are understood as 'environment', from the sitting room in which the interview took place to the faraway land of birth or travel. This layered environment is composed of and indeed requires spaces and places that are varied and thus fragmented and open to different forms of person–place interaction. In the main, our interviews included discussions of places that are engaged spaces, although for most respondents the memory also recalls or explores known places from the past.

We have noted how it is possible to establish for each person an environmental biography that includes their housing history and enables us to consider whether place and space are merely context, or formative in creating, engaging or sustaining identity in later life. This has led us to recognize how people's use of time and space within different types of environment allows them to remain engaged at different levels. The integration of fragmented time and space that enable people to remain relatively autonomous and socially engaged is particularly important and the cross-setting nature of this study has not only brought this to light but has also allowed us to focus on the similarities and differences for people living in mainstream and age-segregated housing in different kinds of location.

The level at which environment affects identity changes over time and for some people it has been greater than for others. However, we acknowledge that as people age, material and social environments can become more visible, more exposed perhaps, as they facilitate or obstruct degrees of engagement, whereas meaning remains essentially interior and personal:

> Well, your home is your base, isn't it? And that's where everything happens, doesn't it? I know you go out and that like, but you always come back don't you, the home is very very important. (Noreen)

References

Age Concern (2003) http://www.ageconcern.org.uk/ageconcern/News_ 1009.htm

Alibhai-Brown, Y. (2000) *Who Do We Think We Are?*, London: Penguin

Altman, I. and Low, S.M. (eds) (1992) *Place Attachment*, New York and London: Plenum Press

Askham, J. (2002) The sociology of ageing in R. Jacoby and C. Oppenheimer (eds) *Psychiatry in the Elderly*, Oxford: Oxford University Press

Baltes, M.M. and Carstensen, L.L. (1996) The process of successful ageing, *Ageing and Society*, 16: pp.397–422

Baltes, P.B. (1997) On the incomplete architecture of human ontogeny: Selection, optimization, and compensation as foundation of developmental theory, *American Psychologist*, 52: pp.366-380

Baltes, P.B. and Baltes, M.M. (1990) Psychological perspectives on successful aging: The model of selective optimization with compensation in P.B. Baltes and M.M. Baltes (eds) *Successful Aging: Perspectives from the behavioural sciences*, New York: Cambridge University Press, pp.1–34

Baltes, P.B. and Mayer, K.U. (eds) (1999) *The Berlin Aging Study: Aging from 70 to 100*, New York: Cambridge University Press

BBC News (2003) Business News, 30/01/03 08:11 GMT, http://news. bbc.co.uk/1/hi/business/2706067.stm

Bic (Boligtrevsel I. Centrum) (1994) Co-housing for senior citizens in Europe, report from EU Conference, *Growing Grey in a Happier Way*, Copenhagen: BiC

Birdwell-Pheasant, D. and Lawrence-Zúñiga, D. (eds) (1999) *House Life-space: Place, space and family in Europe*, Oxford and New York: Berg

Bond, J., Briggs, R. and Coleman, P. (1993) The study of ageing in J. Bond, P. Coleman and S. Peace (eds) *Ageing in Society: An introduction to social gerontology* (2nd edn), London: Sage, pp.29–30

Bornat, J. (1998) 'Working with Life Experience', Block 4, Open University Course K100 *Understanding Health and Social Care*

Bornat, J., Dimmock, B., Jones, D. and Peace, S. (2000) Researching the implications of family-change for older people: The contribution of a life-history approach in P. Chamberlayne, J. Bornat and T. Wengraf (eds) *The Turn of Biographical Methods in Social Science*, London: Routledge, pp.244–260

Bourdieu, P. (1977) *Outline of a Theory of Practice*, Cambridge: Cambridge University Press

Bourdieu, P. (1986) The forms of capital in J. Richardson (ed.) *Handbook of Theory and Research for the Sociology of Education*, New York: Greenwood Press, pp.241–258

Bourdieu, P. and Wacquant, L. (1992) *An Invitation to Reflexive Sociology*, Cambridge: Polity Press

Bowling, A. (2004) *Measuring Health: A review of quality of life measurement scales* (3rd edn), Maidenhead: McGraw-Hill/Open University Press

Breakwell, G.M. (1986) *Coping with Threatened Identities*, London and New York: Methuen

Breakwell, G.M. (1992) *Social Psychology of Identity and the Self-Concept*, London: Surrey University Press and Academic Press Ltd

Breakwell, G.M. (1993) Social representations and social identity, *Papers on Social Representations*, 2(3): pp.2–23

Brenton, M. (2001) Older people's cohousing communities in S. Peace and C. Holland (eds) *Inclusive Housing in an Ageing Society*, Bristol: The Policy Press, pp.169–188

Burkitt, I. (1992) *Social Selves: Theories of the social formation of personality*, London: Sage

Carp, F.M. (1987) Environment and aging in D. Stokols and I. Altman (eds) *Handbook of Environmental Psychology*, New York: Wiley, pp.329–360

Carp, F.M. (1994) Assessing the environment in M.P. Lawton and J.A. Teresi (eds) *Annual Review of Gerontology and Geriatrics* (Vol. 14) New York: Springer, pp.302–323

Carp, F.M. and Carp, A. (1984) A complementary/congruence model of well-being or mental health for the community elderly in I. Altman, M.P. Lawton and J.F. Wohlwill (eds) *Human Behaviour and Environment* (Vol. 7, Elderly people and the environment), New York: Plenum Press, pp.278-336

Chapman, T. and Hockey, J. (eds) (1999) *Ideal Homes?: Social change and domestic life*, London and New York: Routledge

Clapham, D., Means, R. and Munro, M. (1993) Housing, the life course and older people in S. Arber and M. Evandrou (eds) *Ageing, Independence and the Life Course*, London: Jessica Kingsley

Clark, H., Dyer, S. and Horwood, J. (1998) *'That Bit of Help': The high value of low level preventative services for older people*, Bristol: The Policy Press in association with *Community Care* magazine and the Joseph Rowntree Foundation

Clark, William A.V. and Dieleman, F.M. (1996) *Households and Housing: Choice and outcomes in the housing market*, New Brunswick, NJ: Center for Urban Policy and Research

Coleman, P. (1993a) Psychological ageing in P. Coleman, J. Bond and S. Peace (eds) *Ageing in Society: An introduction to social gerontology*, London: Sage, pp.68–96

Coleman, P. (1993b) Adjustment in late life in P. Coleman, J. Bond and S. Peace (eds) *Ageing in Society: An introduction to social gerontology*, London: Sage, pp.97–132

Cooper Marcus, C. (1995) *House as a Mirror of Self: Exploring the deeper meaning of home*, Berkeley, CA: Canari Press

DETR (1998) *English Housing Condition Survey 1996*, London: The Stationery Office

DHSS (1973) *Residential Accommodation for Elderly People*, London: DHSS

Dixon, J.A. and Durrheim, K. (2000). Displacing place identity: A discursive approach to locating self and other, *British Journal of Social Psychology*, 39: pp.27–44

DOE (1975) Housing Single People, Department of the Environment report, London: HMSO

EHCS (1998) *English House Condition Survey 1996*, London: The Stationery Office

ENCC (2003) East Northamptonshire County Council Comprehensive Performance Assessment. Corporate Self-assessment, August 2003, Thrapston: ENC

Erikson, E.H. (1965) *Childhood and Society*. Harmondsworth: Penguin (first published 1950)

Erikson, E.H. (1982) *The Life Cycle Completed: A review*, New York: Norton

Erikson, E.H., Erikson, J.M. and Kivnick, H.Q. (1986) *Vital Involvement in Old Age: The experience of old age in our time*, New York: Norton

Etzioni, A. (1995) *The Spirit of Community: Rights, responsibilities and the communitarian agenda*, London: Fontana

Evandrou, M. and Falkingham, J. (2000) Looking back to look forward: Lessons from four birth cohorts for ageing in the 21st century, *Population Trends*, 99, Spring: pp.27–36

Fisk, M. (2001) The implications of smart home technologies in S. Peace and C. Holland (eds) *Inclusive Housing in an Ageing Society*, Bristol: The Policy Press, pp.101–124

Freud, S. (1917) Mourning and melancholia in J. Strachey (ed.) (1974) *The Standard Edition of the Complete Psychological Works of Sigmund Freud*, London: Hogarth Press

Friedmann, J. (2005) Placemaking as project? Habitus and migration in transnational cities in J. Hillier and E. Rooksby (eds) Habitus: A Sense of Place, London: Ashgate, pp.299–316 Second Edition.

Giddens, A. (1991) *Modernity and Self-Identity*, Cambridge: Polity Press

Glaser, B.G. and Strauss, A. (1967) *The Discovery of Grounded Theory*, Chicago: Aldine

Glaser, K. (1997) The living environments of elderly people, *Reviews in Clinical Gerontology*, 7: pp.63–72

Glaser, K. and Tomassini, C. (2002) Demography in K. Sumner (ed.) *Our Homes, Our Lives: Choice in later life living arrangements*, London: Centre for Policy on Ageing/The Housing Corporation; pp.74–98

Glaser, K., Hancock, R. and Stuchbury, R. (1998) *Attitudes in an Ageing Society* (research sponsored by Age Concern England for the Millennium Debate of the Age), London: Age Concern Institute of Gerontology

Goffman, E. (1959) *The Presentation of Self in Everyday Life*, London: Penguin

Goffman, E. (1961) *Asylums*, London: Penguin

Gregson, N. and Rose, G. (2000) Taking Butler elsewhere: Performativities, spatialities and subjectivities, *Environment and Planning D: Society and Space*, 18: pp.433–452

Grundy, E. (1996) Population review: (5) The population aged 60 and over, *Population Trends*, 84: pp.14–20

Grundy, E. (1999) Intergenerational perspectives on family and household change in mid and later life in England and Wales in S.

McRae (ed.) *Changing Britain. Families and Households in the 1990s*, Oxford: Oxford University Press

Gunter, B. (2000) *Psychology of the Home*, London and Philadelphia: Whurr Publishers

Gurney, C. (1999) Pride and prejudice: Discourses of normalisation in public and private accounts of home ownership, *Housing Studies*, 14(2): pp.163-184

Gurney, C. and Means, R. (1993) The meaning of home in later life in S. Arber and M. Evandrou (eds) *Ageing, Independence and the Life Course*, London: Jessica Kingsley

Gutmann, D.L. (1987) *Reclaimed Powers: Towards a new psychology of men and women in later life*, New York: Basic Books

Hall, E.T. (1966) *The Hidden Dimension*, New York: Doubleday

Hamnett, C. (1991) A nation of inheritors? Housing inheritance, wealth and inequality in Britain, *Journal of Social Policy*, 20(4): pp.504–536

Hanson, J. (2003) *Defining Domesticity: Housing and care choices for older people*, The David Hobman ACIOG Annual Lecture, London: Age Concern and Kings College

Hanson, J., Kellaher, L. and Rowlands, M. (2001) *Profiling the Housing Stock for Older People: The transition from domesticity to caring*, Final Report of EPSRC EQUAL Research, University College London

Hayden, D. (1995) *The Place of Power: Urban landscapes as public history*, Cambridge: MIT Press

Haywood, G. (1977) *Psychological Concepts of Home Among Urban Middle Class Families with Young Children*, City University of New York (unpublished doctoral thesis)

Hediger, H. (1950) *Wild Animals in Captivity*, London: Butterworths

Heywood, F., Pate, E., Means, R. and Galvin, J. (1999) *Housing Options for Older People (Hoop): Report on a developmental project to refine a housing option appraisal tool for use by older people*, London: Elderly Accommodation Council

Heywood, F., Oldman, C. and Means, R. (2002) *Housing and Home in Later Life*, Buckingham: Open University Press

Hillier, B. and Hanson, J. (1984) *The Social Logic of Space*, Cambridge: Cambridge University Press

Hockey, J. and James, A. (2003) *Social Identities across the Life Course*, New York: Palgrave Macmillan

Holland, C. (2001) Housing histories: Older women's experience of home across the life course, Open University (unpublished PhD thesis)

Holland, C., Kellaher, L., Peace, S., Scharf, T., Breeze, E., Gow, J. and Gilhooly, M. (2005) Getting out and about in A. Walker and C.H. Hennessy (eds) *Understanding Quality of Life*. Buckingham: Open University Press, pp.49–63

Holloway, W. and Jefferson, T. (2000) Biography, anxiety and the experience of locality in P. Chamberlayne, J. Bornat and T. Wengraf (eds) *The Turn of Biographical Methods in Social Science*, London: Routledge, pp.167–180

Hormuth, S.E. (1990) *The Ecology of the Self: Relocation and self-concept change*, Cambridge: Cambridge University Press

Jones, C. (1997) The empowerment of older people: Examples of good practice in European countries, Coventry: Community Education Development Centre

Kahana, E. and Kahana, B. (1982) A congruence model of person-environment interaction in M.P. Lawton, P.G. Windley and T.O. Byerts (eds) *Aging and the Environment: Theoretical approaches*, New York: Springer, pp.97–121

Kaplan, R. (1973) Some psychological benefits of gardening, *Environment and Behaviour*, 5(20): pp.145-162

Kaplan, R. (1985) Nature at the doorstep: Residential satisfaction and the nearby environment, *Journal of Architectural Planning Research*, 2: pp.115–127

Kaplan, R. and Kaplan, S. (1987) The garden as a restorative experience in M. Francis and R.T. Hester, Jr (eds) *Meanings of the Garden*, Davis, CA: University of California, pp.334–341

Kaplan, R. and Kaplan, S. (1989) *The Experience of Nature: A psychological perspective*, New York: Cambridge University Press

Katz, J.S. and Peace, S. (2003) *End of Life in Care Homes: A palliative care approach*, Oxford: Oxford University Press

Kaufman, S. (1986) *The Ageless Self – Sources of Meaning in Late Life*, Madison, WI: University of Wisconsin Press

Kaufman, S. (2000) Senescence, decline and the quest for a good death: Contemporary dilemmas and historical antecedents, *Journal of Aging Studies*, 14: pp.1–23

Kellaher, L. (2000) A choice well made: Mutuality as a governing principle in residential care, London: Centre for Policy on Ageing/ Methodist Homes

Kellaher, L. (2002) Is genuine choice a reality?: The range and adequacy of living arrangements available to older people in K. Sumner, *Our Homes, Our Lives: Choice in later life living arrangements*, London: Centre for Policy on Ageing/The Housing Corporation, pp.36–58

Kellaher, L., Peace, S. and Holland, C. (2004) Environment, identity and old age: Quality of life or a life of quality? in A. Walker and C. Hagan Hennessy (eds) *Growing Older: Quality of life in old age*, Maidenhead: Open University Press, pp.60-80

King, R., Warnes, A.M. and Williams, A.M. (2000) *Sunset Lives: British retirement migration to the Mediterranean*, Oxford: Berg

Klatch, R.E. (1999) *A Generation Divided: The New Left, the New Right, and the 1960s.* Berkeley, CA: University of California Press

Koskinen, S. and Outila, M. (2002) Identities, services and quality-of-life. Research programme on ageing in Finland. The village community as a resource for the aged, Elvi-project. BSG Annual Conference 2002, *Active Ageing: Myth or reality?* Birmingham, 12–14 September 2002

Kuo, F.E., Bacaicoas, M. and Sullivan, W.C. (1998) Transforming inner city landscapes: Trees, senses of safety and preference, *Environment and Behaviour*, 30(1): pp.28–59

Laing, W. (2005) *Extra-care Housing Markets 2005*, London: Laing and Buisson

Laws, G. (1997) Spatiality and age relations in A. Jamieson, S. Harper and C. Victor (eds) *Critical Approaches to Ageing and Later Life*, Buckingham: Open University Press

Lawton, M.P. (1980) *Environment and Aging*, Monterey, CA: Brooks/ Cole Publishing Company

Lawton, M.P. (1983) Environment and other determinants of well-being in older people, *The Gerontologist*, 23(4): pp.349–357

Lawton, M.P. (1989) Environmental proactivity in older people in V.L. Bengston and K.W. Schaie (eds) *The Course of Later Life*, New York: Springer, pp.15–23

Lawton, M.P. (1999) Environmental taxonomy: Generalizations from research with older adults in S.L. Friedman and T.D. Wachs (eds) *Measuring Environment across the Life Span*, Washington, DC: American Psychological Association, pp.91–124

Lawton, M.P. and Nahemow, L. (1973) Ecology and the aging process in C. Eisdorpher and M.P. Lawton (eds) *The Psychology of Adult Development and Aging*, Washington, DC: American Psychological Association, pp.619–674

LBH (2003) Haringey Council online Factfile, *http://www.haringey.gov.uk/aboutharingey/fact_file.htm*

Lefebvre, H. (1991) *The Social Production of Space*, Oxford: Blackwell

Lewin, K. (1936) *Principles of Topological Psychology*, New York: McGraw-Hill

Lewis, C.A. (1973) People-plant interaction a new horticultural perspective, *American Horticulturalist*, 52: pp.18-25

Lindberg, E., Garling, T. and Montgomery, H. (1992) Residential-location preferences across the lifespan, *Journal of Environmental Psychology*, 12: pp.187–198

Longhurst, E. (2003) Placing subjectivities, Section 5 in K. Anderson, M. Domosh, S. Pile and N. Thrift (eds) *Handbook of Cultural Geography*, London: Sage, pp.283–289

Low, S.M. (1992) Symbolic ties that bind: Place attachment in the plaza in I. Altman and S. Low (eds) *Place Attachment*, New York: Plenum Press, pp.165–186

Mannheim, K. (1997) The problem of generations in P. Altbach and R. Laufer (eds) *The New Pilgrims: Youth protest in transition*, New York: David McKay and Company, pp.101–138

Marshall, M. (2001) Dementia and technology in S. Peace and C. Holland (eds) *Inclusive Housing in an Ageing Society*, Bristol: The Policy Press

Massey, D. (1994) *Space, Place and Gender*, Cambridge: Polity Press

Mayer, K.U., Maas, I. and Wagner, M. (1999) Socioeconomic conditions and social inequalities in old age in P.B. Baltes and K.U. Mayer (eds) *The Berlin Aging Study: Aging from 70 to 100*, New York: Cambridge University Press, pp.227–255

McCreadie, C. and Tinker, A. (2005) The acceptability of assistive technology to older people, *Ageing & Society*, 25(1): pp.91-110

McGrail, B., Percival, J. and Foster, K. with commentary by Holland, C. and Peace, S. (2001) Integrated segregation? Issues from a range of housing/care environments in S. Peace and C. Holland (eds) *Inclusive Housing in an Ageing Society: Innovative approaches*, Bristol: The Policy Press, pp.147–168

170

Means, R. (1997) Home, independence and community care: Time for a wider vision?, *Policy and Politics*, 25(4): pp.409–420

MHLG (Ministry of Housing and Local Government) (1961) Parker Morris, *Homes for Today and Tomorrow*, London: MHLG

Milligan, M. (1998) Interactional past and potential: The social construction of place attachment, *Symbolic Interaction*, 21, pp.1–3

Mowl, G., Pain, R. and Talbot, C. (2000) The ageing body and the homespace, *Area*, 32: pp.189–197

Mozley, C., Sutcliffe, C., Bagley, H., Cordingley, L., Challis, D., Huxley, P. and Burns, A. (2004) *Towards Quality Care: Outcomes for older people in care homes*, Aldershot: Ashgate

Murphy, M. and Grundy, E. (1994) Co-residence of generations and household structure in Britain: Aspects of change in the 1980s, in H. Becker and P.L.J. Hermkens (eds) *Solidarity of generations: Demographic, economic and social change, and its consequences* (Vol. II), Amsterdam: Thesis Publishers

Murray, H.A. (1938) *Explorations in Personality*, New York: Oxford University Press

Nahemow, L. (2000) The ecological theory of aging: Powell Lawton's legacy in R. Rubinstein, M. Moss and M. Kleban (eds) *The Many Dimensions of Aging*, New York: Springer, pp.22–40

Nasar, J.L. (1989) Perception, cognition and evaluation of urban places in I. Altman and E.H. Zube (eds) *Public Places and Space. Human Behaviour and Environment* (Vol 1), New York: Plenum, pp.31–56

Nasar, J.L., Julian, D., Buchanan, S., Humphrey, D. and Michaly, M. (1983) The emotional quality of scenes and observation points: A look at prospect and refuge, *Landscape Planning*, 10: pp.25–36

National Federation of Housing Associations (1993) Accommodating Diversity: The design of housing for minority ethnic, religious and cultural groups, North Housing Trust, Newcastle upon Tyne.

Newman, O. (1973) *Defensible Space*, New York: Macmillan

ODPM (2001) *Quality and Choice for Older People's Housing – A Strategic Framework*, London: ODPM

Oldman, C. (1990) *Moving in Old Age: New directions in housing policies*, London: HMSO

Oldman, C. and Quilgars, D. (1999) The last resort? Revisiting ideas about older people's living arrangements, *Ageing and Society*, 19(4): pp.363–384

ONS (2002) *Living in Britain – 2001*, London: Office for National Statistics

Park, R.E., Burgess, E.W. and McKenzie, R.D. (1925) *The City*, Chicago: Chicago University Press

Parmelee, P.A. and Lawton, M.P. (1990) The design of special environments for the aged in J.E. Birren and K.W. Schaie (eds) *Handbook of the Psychology of Aging* (3rd edn) San Diego, CA: Academic Press, Inc.: pp.464–488

Peace, S. (1977) *The Elderly in an Urban Environment: A study of spatial mobility in Swansea*, University College Swansea, University of Wales (unpublished PhD thesis)

Peace, S. (1993) The living environments of older women in M. Bernard and K. Meade (eds) *Women Come of Age*, London: Edward Arnold

Peace, S. (2002) The role of older people in research in A. Jamieson and C. Victor (eds) *Researching Ageing and Later Life*, Buckingham: Open University Press, pp.226–244

Peace, S. (forthcoming 2006) 'Housing and Future Living Arrangements' in Vincent, J., Downs, M. and Phillipson, C. (eds) The Futures of Old Age, London: Sage.

Peace, S. and Holland, C. (eds) (2001) *Inclusive Housing in an Ageing Society*, Bristol: The Policy Press

Peace, S., Kellaher, L. and Willcocks, D. (1982) A balanced life: A consumer study of residential life in one hundred local authority old people's homes, Research Report No. 14, Survey Research Unit, London: Polytechnic of North London

Peace, S., Kellaher, L. and Willcocks, D. (1997) *Re-evaluating Residential Care*, Buckingham: Open University Press

Peace, S., Holland, C. and Kellaher, L. (2005) Making space for identity in G.J. Andrews and D.R. Phillips (eds) *Ageing and Place: Perspectives, policy and practice*, Abingdon: Routledge, pp.188–204

Peace, S., Wahl, H.W., Oswald, F. and Mollenkoph, H. (forthcoming, 2006) Environment and ageing: Time, space and place in J. Bond, S. Peace, F. Dittmar-Kohli and G. Westerhof (eds) in *Ageing in Society* (3rd edn), London: Sage

Percival, J. (2000) Gossip in sheltered housing: Its cultural importance and social implications, *Ageing and Society*, 20(3): pp.303–325

Phillips, J., Bernard, M., Biggs, S. and Kingston, P. (2001) Retirement communities in Britain: A 'third way' for a third age? in S. Peace and

C. Holland (eds) *Inclusive Housing in an Ageing Society*, Bristol: The Policy Press, pp.189-214

Phillipson, C. (2004) Urbanization and ageing: towards a new environmental gerontology, review article, *Ageing and Society*, 24(6): pp.963–972

Phillipson, C., Bernard, M., Phillips, J. and Ong, M. (2001) *The Family and Community Life of Older People: Social networks and social support in three urban areas*, London: Routledge

Pile, S. and Thrift, N. (eds) (1995) *Mapping the Subject: Geographies of cultural transformation*, London: Routledge

Popular Housing Forum (1998) Kerb appeal: The external appearance and site layout of new houses, Report Number 1, UK: Popular Housing Forum

Probyn, E. (2003) The spatial imperative of subjectivity in K. Anderson, M. Domosh, S. Pile and N. Thrift (eds) (2003) *Handbook of Cultural Geography*, London: Sage, pp.290–299

Rapoport, A. (1969) *House Form and Culture*, Englewood Cliffs, NJ: Prentice-Hall

Ratcliffe, P. (1999) Housing inequality and 'Race': Some critical reflections on the concept of 'social exclusion', *Ethnic and Racial Studies*, 22(1), pp.1-22

Riggs, A. and Turner, B.S. (2000) Pie-eyed optimists: Baby boomers the optimistic generation?, *Social Indicators Research*, 52: pp.73-93

Rohde, C.L.E. and Kendle, A.D. (1994) *Human Well-being, Natural Landscapes and Wildlife in Urban Areas: A review*, Reading: University of Reading for English Nature

Rossi, P. (1955) *Why Families Move: A study in the social psychology of residential mobility*, Glencoe, MI: Free Press

Rowles, G.D. (1978) *Prisoners of Space/Exploring the Geographic Experience of Older People*, Boulder, CO: Westview

Rowles, G.D. (1981) The surveillance zone as meaningful space for the aged, *Gerontologist*, 21(3): pp.304–311

Rowles, G.D. (1983) Place and personal identity in old age: Observations from Appalachia, *Journal of Environmental Psychology*, 3: pp.299–313

Rowles, G.D. (1991) Beyond performance: Being in place as a component of occupational therapy, *American Journal of Occupational Therapy*, 45: pp.111–130

Rowles, G.D. (2000) Habituation and being in place, *Occupational Therapy Journal of Research*, 20 (Supplement): pp.52S–67S

Rowles, G.D. and Watkin, J.F. (2003) History, habit, heart and hearth: on making spaces into places in K.W. Schaie, H.W. Wahl, H. Mollenkopf and F. Oswald (eds) *Aging Independently: Living arrangements and mobility*, New York: Springer

Rowles, G.D., Oswald, F. and Hunter, E. (2004) Interior living environments in old age in H.W. Wahl, R.J. Scheidt and P.G. Windley (eds) *Aging in Context: socio-physical environments, Annual Review of Gerontology and Geriatrics* (Vol. 23), New York: Springer, pp.167–194

Rubinstein, R.L. (1989) The home environments of older people: A description of the psycho-social processes linking person to place, *Journal of Gerontology: Social Sciences*, pp.44–56

Rubinstein, R.L. (1990) Personal identity and environmental meaning in later life, *Journal of Aging Studies*, 4: pp.131–148

Rubinstein, R.L. and De Medeiros, K. (2004) Ecology and the aging self in H.W. Wahl, R.J. Scheidt and P.G. Windley (eds) *Aging in Context: Socio-physical environments, Annual Review of Gerontology and Geriatrics* (Vol. 23), New York: Springer, pp.59–84

Rubinstein, R.L. and Parmelee, P. (1992) Attachment to place and the representation of the life course by the elderly in I. Altman and S.M. Low (eds) *Place Attachment*, New York and London: Plenum Press, pp.139–163

Saunders, P. (1990) *A Nation of Home Owners*, London: Unwin Hyman

Saunders, P. and Williams, P. (1988) The constitution of the home: Towards a research agenda, *Housing Studies*, 3(2): pp.91-93

Shlay, A.B. (1985) Castles in the sky: Measuring housing and neighbourhood ideology, *Environment and Behaviour*, 17(5): pp.593–626

Sixsmith, A. (1986) The meaning of home: An exploratory study of environmental experience, *Journal of Environmental Psychology*, 6: pp.281–298

Sixsmith, A. (1990) The meaning and experience of 'home' in later life in B. Bytheway and J. Johnson (eds) *Welfare and the Ageing Experience*, Aldershot: Avebury

Smith, J., Fleeson, W., Geiselmann, B., Settersten, R.S. Jr and Kunzmann, U. (1999) Sources of well-being in very old age in P.B. Baltes and K.U. Mayer (eds) *The Berlin Aging Study: Aging from 70 to 100*,

New York: Cambridge University Press, pp.450–471

Soja, E. (1989) *Postmodern Geographies*, London: Verso

Sommer, R. (1969) *Personal Space: The behavioural basis of design*, Englewood Cliffs, NJ: Prentice-Hall, Inc.

Staudinger, U.M., Freund, A.M., Linden, M. and Maas, I. (1999) Self, personality, and life regulation: Facets of psychological resilience in old age in P.B. Baltes and K.U. Mayer (eds) *The Berlin Aging Study: Aging from 70 to 100*, New York: Cambridge University Press, pp.302–328

Steinfeld, E. (1981) The place of old age: The meaning of housing for old people in J. Duncan (ed.) *Housing and Identity: Cross-cultural perspectives*, London; Croom Helm, pp.198–246

Strauss, A. (1987) *Qualitative Analysis for Social Scientists*, Cambridge: Cambridge University Press

Sugarman, L. (1986) *Life-span Development: Concepts, theories and interventions*, London: Methuen

Sumner, K. (2002) *Our Homes, Our Lives: Choice in later life living arrangements*, London: Centre for Policy on Ageing/The Housing Corporation

Taylor, M., Barr, A. and West, A. (2000) *Signposts to Community Development* (2nd edn), London: CDF Publications

Taylor, R.B. and Brower, S.D. (1985) Home and near-home territories in I. Altman and C.M. Werner, *Home Environments*, New York: Plenum Press, pp.1–32

Toffaleti, C. (1997) *The Older People's Initiative: Giving older people a say – acting locally to improve housing choices*, Greater Manchester: CVO

Townsend, P. (1962) *The Last Refuge – A Survey of Residential Institutions and Homes for the Aged in England and Wales*. London: Routledge & Kegan Paul

Tuan, Yi-Fu (1974) *Topophilia: A Study of Environmental Perception, Attitudes and Values*, New York: Columbia University Press

Twigg, J. (1999) The spatial ordering of care: Public and private in bathing support at home, *Sociology of Health and Illness*, 21: pp.381–400

Twigger-Ross, C.L. and Uzzell, D.L. (1996) Place and identity processes, *Journal of Environmental Psychology*, 16: pp.206–220

Ulrich, R.S., Simons, R.F., Losito, B.D., Fiorito, E., Miles, M.A. and Zelson, M. (1991) Stress recovery during exposure to nature and urban environment, *Journal of Environmental Psychology*, 11: pp.201–236

Veitch, R. and Arkkelin, D. (1995) *Environmental Psychology: An interdisciplinary perspective*, Englewood Cliffs, NJ: Prentice-Hall, Inc.

VROM (Ministerie van Volkshuisvesting, Ruimtelijke Ordening en Milieubeheer) (1997) *Huisvesting van Ouderen op het Breukvlak van twee Eeuwen*, Zoetermeer: VROM

Wahl, H.W. (2003) Research on living arrangements in old age for what? In K. Warner-Schaie, H.-W. Wahl, H. Mollenkopf and F. Oswald (eds) *Aging Independently: Living arrangements and mobility*, New York: Springer

Wahl, H.W. and Lang, F.R. (2004) Aging in context across the adult life course: Integrating physical and social environmental research perspective in H.W. Wahl, R.J. Scheidt and P.G. Windley (eds) *Aging in context: Socio-physical environments, Annual Review of Gerontology and Geriatrics* (Vol. 23), New York: Springer, pp.1–33

Walker, A. and Hagan Hennessy, C. (2005) *Understanding Quality of Life in Old Age*, Maidenhead: McGraw-Hill/Open University Press

Warnes, A. (1991) Migration to and seasonal residences in Spain of northern European elderly people, *European Journal of Gerontology and Geriatrics*, 1: pp.185–194

Warnes, A. (1996) Migrations among older people, reviews, *Clinical Gerontology*, 6: pp.101–114

Warnes, A. (ed) (2004) Older Migrants in Europe: Essays, Projects and Sources, Sheffield: Sheffield Institute for Studies on Ageing.

Watt, P. (1993) Housing inheritance and social inequality: A rejoinder to Chris Hamnett, *Journal of Social Policy*, 22(4): pp.527–534

Wetherall, M. (ed.) (1996) *Identities, Groups and Social Issues*, London: Sage

WHO (2000) Quality of life: A consensus document, WHO-IASSID Work Plan, prepared by The Special Interest Research Group on Quality of Life, August 2000

Willcocks, D., Peace, S. and Kellaher, L. (1987) *Private Lives in Public Places*, London: Tavistock Publications

Index

Page numbers in *italics* refer to figures.